临床操作专业英语

Professional English for Clinical Practice

主　　编　胡亚南　毛　帅

主　　审　张敏州

副 主 编　张晓璇　何健卓　王芳芳

英文审校　**Prof. Aleksander Hinek　Dr. Alice Kiger**
Terra Hyland

编　　委（按姓氏笔画排序）

王　芸　新疆医科大学
王芳芳　广东省中医院
毛　帅　广东省中医院
刘晓杰　山东中医药大学
安雪梅　黑龙江中医药大学
孙瑞丽　山西中医药大学
何健卓　广东省中医院
张晓璇　广东省中医院
张建东　广州中医药大学第一附属医院
陈　战　山东中医药大学
周　芬　北京中医药大学
赵晓燕　安徽中医药大学
胡亚南　广州中医药大学
袁　娟　安徽中医药大学
解　东　长春中医药大学
谭益冰　广州中医药大学
潘兰霞　河南中医药大学

人民卫生出版社

图书在版编目（CIP）数据

临床操作专业英语 / 胡亚南，毛帅主编 . —北京：人民卫生出版社，2017

ISBN 978-7-117-25675-9

Ⅰ. ①临⋯　Ⅱ. ①胡⋯ ②毛⋯　Ⅲ. ①临床医学 - 英语　Ⅳ. ①R4

中国版本图书馆 CIP 数据核字（2017）第 301091 号

| 人卫智网 | www.ipmph.com | 医学教育、学术、考试、健康，购书智慧智能综合服务平台 |
| 人卫官网 | www.pmph.com | 人卫官方资讯发布平台 |

临床操作专业英语

主　　编：胡亚南　毛 帅
出版发行：人民卫生出版社（中继线 010-59780011）
地　　址：北京市朝阳区潘家园南里 19 号
邮　　编：100021
E - mail：pmph @ pmph.com
购书热线：010-59787592　010-59787584　010-65264830
印　　刷：三河市博文印刷有限公司
经　　销：新华书店
开　　本：787×1092　1/16　印张：8
字　　数：175 千字
版　　次：2018 年 2 月第 1 版　2018 年 2 月第 1 版第 1 次印刷
标准书号：ISBN 978-7-117-25675-9/R・25676
定　　价：38.00 元

打击盗版举报电话：010-59787491　E-mail: WQ @ pmph.com
（凡属印装质量问题请与本社市场营销中心联系退换）

序言

近年来,随着国际交流的不断增加,中国的临床医学水平得到了突飞猛进的发展,同时外籍患者的人数亦迅速增加。在世界医学平台上与同行进行全方位的交流,在涉外诊疗工作中准确、详尽地表达医务人员的意见,这是许多临床医务工作者迫切需要的。

要达到这个目的,对于大多数中国医生、护士而言,语言是一个需要解决的主要问题。不仅要掌握好英语,而且要掌握好医学英语,这是一项需要付出长期努力的工作,不是一朝一夕就可以完成的。但我们并不怕困难,关键是要正视困难。

临床医学(clinical medicine)是医学中侧重实践活动的部分,是直接面对疾病、患者,对患者直接实施治疗的科学。临床医护人员需要掌握涉及内、外、妇、儿等多学科的广博医学知识及专业用语,这更是对专业英语提出了具体的要求,而目前专门针对临床操作的专业英语著作仍相对缺乏。为帮助广大临床医务工作者和医学生学习英语,迅速掌握临床英语会话,几位有国外医学留学经历及国内从事临床一线工作的医生、护士们一起编写了《临床操作专业英语》。

通过对《临床操作专业英语》的学习,医生、护士们可以学会如何与病人在所有领域内进行有效交流:包括从踏入医院,到接诊问诊、进行各项检测和身体检查,住院观察和出院手续办理等。同时,本书特别列举出临床医学各科常用的英语单词及短语,以利于学习者归纳总结。

本书具有以下特点:

1. 力求实用 使学习者在掌握语言技能的同时,能够在模拟诊疗的环境中操练英语交际技能,了解和巩固相关的医学知识。

2. 具有针对性 语言素材的选择符合从医人员和相关学习者的特点和实际水平,并充分考虑到从医人员面对外籍患者可能产生的表达困难,从关键且容易理解的医学背景知识切入主题,从不同角度举一反三地操练听说技能,提高其医疗英语的应用能力。

3. 涵盖多元文化 《临床操作专业英语》提供的各类医疗文化场景将帮助医务人员正确面对和处理外籍患者所注重的文化和传统观念。

《临床操作专业英语》简单实用,不仅适用于医学院校的师生、从事临床医学专业的在职医护人员,同样对在医院就诊的患者及其家属来说也是一本必备的指导手册。

千里之行,始于足下。希望本书能够帮助临床医学各专业的医务工作者有效地提高专业英语水平,有助于他们在国际医学学术交流和涉外诊疗活动中更出色地发挥专业优势。由此,我谨向大家推荐本书。

管向东

中山大学附属第一医院

2017 年 10 月

前言

　　随着国际交流的日益增多,越来越多的中国医务工作者走出了国门,走向了国际。同时国内的医务工作者也有了越来越多的机会接诊到外籍人士,英语作为一种国际通用语言,无论在护理患者还是在与患者沟通交流病情上都起到了非常重要的作用。目前市面上大部分的医学类专业英语书籍,包括医疗、护理的专业英语教材,大多以国外(英美为主)的医疗环境作为背景开展技能活动。这类书籍更多地适用于准备出国学习或就业的医护人员选用,而针对在本国内的医疗场景中如何使用专业英语开展相关技能活动,这一类的书籍是相对欠缺的。这里主要的一个原因是对专业英语在使用过程中准确性的把握有一定难度。有英语背景的人通常没有专业的医疗知识,有医疗背景的人又没有专业的英语水平。为保证国内医疗场景中英语应用的地道及准确性,我们在本书修稿过程中邀请了三位来自英、美国家医疗护理领域的专家进行审稿,其中一位美籍专家同时拥有中文 HSK 五级证书,故此保障了英语使用的准确性。本书的编写适应当前医学教育的改革与发展趋势,在强化实践技能的过程中,提升准确使用英语表达的能力,满足国际化发展的需要。本书从构思到编写都以高标准要求,力求全书结构体例规范,编写风格一致,内容科学严谨。

　　《临床操作专业英语》一书共分为27章,内容涉及医疗护理活动中常见的技能操作。每章由三大部分组成:第一部分是背景介绍。如患者的病情,操作技术相关知识点的介绍;第二部分是在具体的技能操作场景中英语的使用,以对话的形式呈现,力求体现实用性,准确性及易读性的特点;第三部分是相关专业词汇的学习及例句的分析。

　　本书的编委来自全国各大高校及临床一线的医护人员,大部分编委老师参与了"十三五"规划教材《护理专业英语》的编写,具有丰富的临床及编写经验。本书可供我国高等医学及护理学专业的学生使用,也可供从事医学相关专业的教学工作者,及临床一线的医护人员使用和参考。

　　本书在编写过程中得到了各位老师及专家的大力支持,张敏州教授作为主审给予了很多宝贵的指导性意见,在此一并表示诚挚的感谢。本书全体编者都以高度认真负责的态度参与了工作,但因各医院及高校实际情况的差异,少许偏差在所难免,敬请各院校师生、临床医护工作者在使用本书过程中,提出意见和建议,以求修订时改进与完善。希望本书的出版,能够对全国医疗护理专业的师生及一线临床工作者使用英语产生积极的推动作用。

胡亚南　毛　帅

2017 年 10 月

目录

CONTENTS

Chapter One Admission

第一章
入　院

Part One Case Presentation

Mrs. Zhang, a 48-year-old female was admitted in the Emergency Department of a general hospital at 1: 40 a.m. on June 30, 2015. She had suffered a **blunt head trauma** from a traffic accident. She took some blood tests and a CT scan upon admission. CT findings indicated that she had a **contusion**. Her **vital signs** were not very **stable**. Her **oxygen saturations** upon admission were 90%. She was on 4 liters of oxygen (O_2) at that time. IV drip was set up and primary **disposal** of the wound was done. She was immediately sent to the **Intensive Care Unit** (ICU) for further **observation** and **treatment**.

第一部分　病案介绍

张女士,48 岁,女性,于 2015 年 6 月 30 日凌晨 1 点 40 分由于车祸急诊入院某综合性医院急诊科。入院后马上进行血液检查和脑部 CT 扫描。脑部 CT 结果表明患者患有脑挫裂伤。患者生命体征不稳定,入院时血氧饱和度为 90%,给予吸氧每分钟 4 升,静脉输液,基本的伤口处理。为进一步观察病情和治疗将患者紧急送往重症监护室。

Part Two Dialogue

第二部分　对　话

Nurse: Hello, Mrs. Zhang? I am your bed nurse, Liu Yang. Can you open your eyes, please?
护士:张女士您好,我是您的责任护士,我叫刘洋。您能睁开眼睛吗?

Mrs. Zhang: Urgh.

张女士：啊。

Nurse: That's it. Do you know where you are?

护士：您知道您在哪吗?

Mrs. Zhang: I am not sure where I am.

张女士：我不太清楚。

Nurse: You are in the ICU of the hospital. You've had a head injury from a traffic accident. How are you feeling now?

护士：您在医院的重症监护室。由于车祸导致头部受伤。您现在感觉怎么样?

Mrs. Zhang: Cold.

张女士：冷。

Nurse: I will get you a blanket, you will feel better.

护士：我给您拿条毯子吧,那样会好些。

Mrs. Zhang: Mm.

张女士：嗯。

Nurse: Are you in any pain?

护士：您感觉哪里疼吗?

Mrs. Zhang: Mm ... no.

张女士：不。

Nurse: That's good. We administered a **painkiller** to you before you left the Emergency Department.

护士：好的。刚才在急诊科给您有用过止痛剂。

Nurse: Hello, who are you?

护士：您好,您是哪位?

Mr. Zhou: Hello, I am her husband. How is she?

周先生：我是患者的丈夫,我妻子怎么样了?

Nurse: I'm just going to take her vital signs again. This is Dr. Wang, one of the most experienced surgeons in the hospital. He is in charge of your wife.

护士：我需要再观察一下她的病情。这位是刘医生,我院最有经验的外科医生之一,他是您妻子的主治医生。

Dr. Liu: Hello, I will give you a thorough explanation about her conditions later, now I am examining her. OK?

刘医生：您好,我稍后会详细介绍您妻子的病情,现在我先给她做检查,好吗?

Mr. Zhou: All right.

周先生：好的。

Nurse: Mr. Zhou, let me tell you some rules in our ICU. Your family can not stay with her in the ICU, but we have visiting hours.

护士: 周先生,我给您介绍一下患者在重症监护室住院的相关事项。您的家人不能待在监护室内,不过,会给探视的时间。

Mr. Zhou: When shall we visit?

周先生: 什么时间可以探视?

Nurse: Visiting hours are from 1 p.m. to 2 p.m. and from 6 p.m. to 7 p.m. Only two visitors are allowed to enter the ICU each time. Would you like to tell me your cell phone number so that we can inform you about the patient's conditions at any time? (Please be sure that your cell phone is turned on 24 hours a day.)

护士: 探视时间是下午 1 至 2 点,晚上 6 至 7 点。不过每次只允许两名家属进入监护室。您可以留一下联系方式吗? 以便我们告知(沟通)患者病情(请务必保持手机 24 小时畅通)。

Mr. Zhou: OK, and what should she do if she needs help?

周先生: 好的。如果她需要帮助,怎么办?

Nurse: (The nurse turns to the patient and says) Mrs. Zhang, can you hear me? The headboard by the bedside is equipped with a calling system. If you need any help, please press the button. In any case, the nurse will be 24 hours to monitor your condition.

护士:(护士转向患者)张女士,您可以听见我说话吗? 如果您需要护士的帮助,床头案板上装有呼叫系统,您按床旁按钮就可以的。不管怎样,护士会 24 小时监护您的病情。

Mr. Zhou: OK, I see. What about the meal time?

周先生: 我知道了。您能说一下就餐时间吗?

Nurse: The meal time is 7 a.m. for breakfast, 12 at noon for lunch, and 6 p.m. for dinner. I don't think she can eat now, we just started her **intravenous infusion** according the doctor's orders.

护士: 早餐是 7 点开始,午餐是 12 点,晚餐是 6 点。我想她现在不能进食,我们遵照医嘱给予了静脉输液。

Mr. Zhou: Thank you so much.

周先生: 非常感谢。

Nurse: You are welcome. Dr. Liu will talk to you about her condition later.

护士: 不客气。稍后,刘医生会向您介绍您妻子的病情。

Part Three　Words and Phrases

第三部分　单词和短语

contusion [kən'tjuːʒ(ə)n] *n.* 挫伤

【例句】The clinical data of 36 cases of severe pulmonary contusion were reviewed. 对 36 例

严重肺挫伤患者的临床资料进行回顾性分析。

stable ['steɪb(ə)l] *adj.* 稳定的

【例句】The patient's condition is stable and not life-threatening. 病人的状况稳定,不会危及生命。

blunt [blʌnt] *adj.* 钝的;生硬的 blunt head trauma 头钝器伤

trauma ['traʊmə] *n.* [外科]创伤

【例句】Blunt head trauma can happen from a blow to the head, and result in serious damage to the brain. 打击头部引起头部钝器伤的发生,能够导致严重的脑损伤。

oxygen ['ɒksɪdʒ(ə)n] *n.* 氧气

saturation [sætʃə'reɪʃ(ə)n] *n.* 饱和度

【例句】Monitoring arterial oxygen saturation in the blood becomes more and more important in clinical medicine. 在临床医学中,监测动脉血氧饱和度越来越重要。

disposal [dɪ'spəʊz(ə)l] *n.* 处理

【例句】Now people pay more attention to the environment pollution problems, which are caused by inappropriate disposal of medical waste. 现在人们更加注意由不恰当的处理医用垃圾所引起的环境污染问题。

monitor ['mɒnɪtə] *v.* 监控;监听;监测 *n.* 监控器

【例句】The instrument monitors the patient's heartbeats. 仪器监护病人的心跳。

observation [ɒbzə'veɪʃ(ə)n] *n.* 观察

【例句】This result must be confirmed by further experimental study and clinical observation. 这个(试验)结果必须通过进一步的试验研究和临床观察来证实。

treatment ['triːtm(ə)nt] *n.* 治疗

【例句】Her illness is not responding to the new treatment. 新疗法对她的病无效。

painkiller *n.* 止痛药

【例句】Objective to observed the effects of painkiller combined with sedatives were continually used in acute myocardial infarction (AMI) patients. 目的是观察急性心肌梗死(AMI)患者的止痛药跟镇静药联合治疗的效果。

intravenous [ˌɪntrə'viːnəs] *adj.* 静脉内的

infusion [ɪn'fjuːʒ(ə)n] *n.* 输液;输注;灌输;浸泡

intravenous infusion 静脉输液

【例句】Intravenous infusions are used when patients need medications, fluids, electrolytes, or nutritional supplements that can not be taken orally. 静脉输液用于病人需要药物、液体、电解质或营养物质补充而不能经口摄入的情况。

medication [medɪ'keɪʃ(ə)n] *n.* 药物;药物治疗

concussion [kən'kʌʃ(ə)n] *n.* 脑震荡

cranial ['kreɪnɪəl] *adj.* 颅骨的

cranioplasty ['kreɪnɪəˌplæstɪ] *n.* 颅骨成形术

cerebral ['serɪbr(ə)l] *adj.* 大脑的

【例句】They found that white opaque patches and whitened blood vessels on the retina were unique signs of cerebral malaria. 他们发现视网膜上的白色不透明斑点和变成白色的血管是脑疟疾的独特标志。

hemorrhage ['hɛmərɪdʒ] *n.* [病理]出血（等于 haemorrhage）；番茄汁 *vt.* [病理]出血 *vi.* [病理]出血

【例句】Your patient has suffered a type of stroke called subarachnoid hemorrhage (SAH). 您的病人患上了一种名为蛛网膜下出血（SAH）的中风症。

cerebrovascular [ˌserɪbrə(ʊ)'væskjʊlə] *adj.* 脑血管的

hydrocephalus [ˌhaɪdrə'sef(ə)ləs] *n.* 脑积水

encephalopathy [enˌsefə'lɒpəθɪ] *n.* 脑病

intubation [ˌɪntju: 'beɪʃən] *n.* [临床]插管 endotracheal intubation 气管内插管

extubation [ˌekstju: 'beɪʃən] *n.* 拔管

consciousness ['kɒnʃəsnɪs] *n.* 意识

CT scan   计算机横断面扫描（computerized tomography）

MRI   核磁共振（magnetic resonance imaging）

ICU   重症监护室（intensive care unit）

Phrases and Expressions

in charge of   负责；主管
be equipped with   装用…装置；装备有

（解　东）

第二章
生命体征监测

Part One   Case Presentation

Mrs. Lin, 65 years old, hospitalized with chest pain for two hours, has been diagnosed with **acute myocardial infarction (AMI)**. She has **radiating** pain in her left shoulder and **squeezing** chest pain. She took some painkillers at home, but that didn't relieve her symptoms. She also feels **nauseated** and vomited a few times before **hospitalization**. She took one **nitroglycerin** tablet half an hour ago, but that didn't work either. She is **sweating**. In order to collect more information to have an overall understanding of the patient's situation, the charge nurse is going to take her vital signs, and below is their conversation.

第一部分   病案介绍

林女士,65 岁,因胸闷痛 2 小时入院,诊断为急性心肌梗死。病人主诉胸闷痛及左肩部放射痛,病人在家里自行服用了一些止痛药但是并没有缓解疼痛。病人觉得恶心,入院前已经呕吐过数次。半小时前含服了一粒硝酸甘油,目前还没有起效,病人在不停冒汗。为了收集更多的信息以便对病人的病情有更全面的了解,管床护士将要对病人的生命体征进行监测,以下是她们的对话。

Part Two   Dialogue

第二部分   对   话

Nurse: Hello, Mrs. Lin. I'm your charge nurse, Sun Hong. You can call me Xiao Sun if you want. I need to check your vital signs. It will take about 15 minutes, is that OK?

护士：你好,林女士,我是您的主管护士孙红,您可以叫我小孙。我需要监测您的生命体征。大概需要 15 分钟,可以吗？

Mrs. Lin: Hello, Xiao Sun, that's OK, but what are **vital signs** exactly?

林女士：你好,小孙,可以的,但是什么是生命体征？

Nurse: Vital signs are your temperature, heart rate, **respiratory** rate and blood pressure.

护士：生命体征是指您的体温、心率、呼吸以及血压。

Mrs. Lin: OK, I see。

林女士：好的,我知道了。

Nurse: Firstly, I need to attach these **electrodes** to your skin。

护士：首先,我需要把这些电极片贴到你身体表面。

Nurse: Secondly, I need to take your blood pressure.

护士：其次,我需要测一下您的血压。

Nurse: Now, please put this on your finger, it will help to check your oxygen saturation. And I'll put this **thermometer** in your **armpit** to take your temperature.

护士：现在,请将这个戴在手指上,这个是帮助我们监测您的血氧饱和度。体温计放到腋窝监测体温。

Mrs. Lin: How are my vital signs?

林女士：我的生命体征怎么样？

Nurse: Your heart rate is 85 beats per minute; blood pressure is one fifty-five over ninety-seven mmHg, which is higher than normal; your respiration rate is 22 times per minute; let me check your temperature, umm, it's thirty-seven degrees, it's normal.

护士：你的心率是 85 次 / 分钟；血压是 155/97mmHg,比正常会高一些；呼吸是 22 次 / 分钟；让我看下你的体温,是 37 度,正常的。

Nurse: Okay, I've finished. Don't worry too much, we will take care of you. Is there anything else I can do for you?

护士：好了我做完了,不要太担心了,我们会照顾您的,还有什么事需要我帮忙吗？

Mrs. Lin: I still feel nauseated and sweating, can you give me some medication?

林女士：我还是觉得有点儿恶心,不停地出汗,你可以给我吃点儿药吗？

Nurse: I will report that to your doctor, and here is your call light, if you need anything before I come back, please ring the bell.

护士：我会把这个情况汇报给您的主治医生,这里有个呼叫铃,如果在我回来之前您有任何需要,请随时按铃。

Mrs. Lin: That's very helpful, thank you very much.

林女士：这个很有帮助,非常感谢你!

Nurse: You are welcome, see you soon.

护士: 不客气,马上回来。

Part Three　Words and Phrases

第三部分　单词和短语

myocardial [ˌmaɪəˈkɑːrdɪəl] *adj.* 心肌的

infarction [ɪnˈfɑːrkʃən] *n.* 梗塞;[病理]梗塞形成,梗死形成

acute myocardial infarction (AMI) 急性心肌梗死

【例句】To assess the value of percutaneous coronary intervention (PCI) on patients with acute myocardial infarction (AMI). 目的探讨急性心肌梗塞(AMI)急诊经皮冠状动脉介入治疗(PCI)的治疗价值。

vital [ˈvaɪtl] *adj.* 至关重要的;生死攸关的;有活力的

vital sign 生命体征

【例句】It is vital that parents give children clear and consistent messages about drugs. 至关重要的是,父母要给孩子们明确一致的关于药物的信息。

radiating [ˈreɪdɪeɪtɪŋ] *adj.* 发射出(光、热等)(radiate 的现在分词)*v.*(使品质或情感)显出,流露;射出,向四周伸出;散热

【例句】If you've noticed a sudden shooting pain radiating from your buttocks and traveling down one leg, it's probably that pesky uterus as well, flattening your sciatic nerve. 如果突然出现从臀部至单侧腿的放射疼痛,那很可能就是子宫在压迫你的坐骨神经。

squeezing [skˈwiːzɪŋ] *adj.* 挤压的;压榨的

【例句】It is taking decisions whose consequences are not only squeezing the middle class, but threatening its very existence. 政府所做的决定不但是在压榨中产阶级,还在危及整个阶级的存在。

nauseate [ˈnɔːzɪet] *vi.* 作呕;厌恶;产生恶感 *vt.* 使厌恶;使恶心;使作呕

【例句】She could not eat anything without feeling nauseated. 吃任何东西她都会感到恶心

sweating [ˈswetɪŋ] *v.* 出汗(sweat 的 ing 形式)*n.* 发汗(等于 exudation)

【例句】We aren't a bit afraid of bleeding and sweating. 我们一点也不害怕流血和流汗。

electrode [ɪˈlɛktrod] *n.* 电极

【例句】With this new tool, you can determine exactly where to place the stimulation electrode in the brain. 有了新工具,你就可以准确地确定把刺激电极放置在大脑的哪个位置。

thermometer [θɚˈmɑmɪtɚ] *n.* 温度计;体温计

【例句】Put this thermometer under you tongue. 把这个温度计放在你的舌头下面。

armpit ['ɑrm'pɪt] *n.* 腋窝

【例句】There are some swellings in his armpit. 他的腋窝下有些肿大的部分。

hospitalization [ˌhɑːspɪtələˈzeɪʃn] *n.* 住院治疗；医院收容；住院保险（等于 hospitalization insurance）

【例句】The doctor advised hospitalization for the child. 医生建议给孩子住院治疗。

nitroglycerin ['naɪtrəˈglɪsərɪn] *n.* 硝酸甘油；硝化甘油

【例句】Average weekly use of nitroglycerin tablets to fight chest pain fell from 55 to 2 in the same period. 在同一时期，平均每周使用硝酸甘油药片治疗胸痛的时间从 55 减少到 2。

respiratory [rɪˈspaɪərətɔːrɪ] *adj.* 呼吸的

【例句】Authorities also are watching for respiratory illnesses, such as the common cold, influenza and tuberculosis. 当局还在密切关注呼吸道疾病，如普通感冒、流感和肺结核。

Phrases and Expressions

frequency of　……频率

the former　前者

（胡亚南）

Chapter Three   Physical Examination

第三章
体格检查

Part One   Case Presentation

Mr. Li, a 48-year-old male, is hospitalized with right-side chest pain accompanied by palpitation and difficulty breathing when lifting up heavy items, and is diagnosed with spontaneous **pneumothorax**. He complains of a sudden stinging of pain on the right **thorax**, **palpitation**, a choking **sensation** in his chest and difficulty breathing. He also has irritable dry coughing and has a cold sweat over his whole body. The symptoms remain even after taking a rest. In order to collect more information to have an overall knowledge about his condition, the doctor is going to carry out a physical examination. The following is their conversation.

第一部分   病 案 介 绍

李先生,48 岁,抬重物时突发右侧胸痛,伴心悸、呼吸困难入院。诊断为自发性气胸。病人主诉右胸突然针刺样疼痛,心悸、胸闷、呼吸困难,有刺激性干咳,全身冷汗,休息后未缓解。为了收集更多的信息以更全面地了解他的病情,医生将要对他进行体格检查。以下是他们的对话。

Part Two   Dialogue

第二部分   对   话

Doctor: Hello, Mr. Li. I'm the doctor in charge of your case. To make a definitive diagnosis, you need to have an overall physical examination. It will take about half an hour, is that OK?

医生:您好! 李先生,我是您的主管医生,为了明确诊断,我需要给您做一次全面的体格检查,大约需要 30 分钟的时间,可以吗?

Mr. Li: OK, I will try my best to cooperate.

病人:好的,我会尽量配合您的。

Doctor: Since the nurse has checked your vital signs just now, I will move on to other examinations for you.

医生:刚刚护士已经监测过您的生命体征,接下来我将为您做其他检查。

Doctor: First, I will check your head. I need to check your eyes with a small light, please take it easy. Now please fix your gaze on my finger, and move your eyeballs with it. Well done. Now let me check your ears, nose, and mouth.

医生:首先检查一下您的头部。我需要用手电筒检查一下您的眼睛,不用紧张。现在请您注视我的手指,眼球跟随我的手指运动。很好,现在我来检查一下您的耳、鼻、口。

Mr. Li: Anything wrong with me?

李先生:有什么问题吗?

Doctor: Nothing so far. I will check your neck.

医生:目前为止没什么问题。我再检查一下您的颈部。

Doctor: The movements are normal. There are no swollen **lymph** nodes. The **thyroid** gland is not swollen, but the **trachea** sways to the left slightly.

医生:颈部活动正常。没有肿大的淋巴结。甲状腺不肿大,但是气管略向左偏。

Doctor: Now, I will use the **stethoscope** to listen to your heart. Good! There is no **vascular murmur**.

医生:现在,我用听诊器听一下心脏。很好,颈部没有血管杂音。

Mr. Li: Any other checks?

李先生:还有其他检查吗?

Doctor: Yes. Please unbutton your jacket, and expose fully your chest and abdomen. Well, let me check there.

医生:是的。请你解开上衣,充分暴露胸、腹部。让我检查一下。

Doctor: The **bilateral** breasts are **symmetric**, the skin is normal, and the **cardiac** impulse is regular. There is no **anomalous upheaval** in your **precordium**. However, the right thorax is swollen. It is weakening the respiratory movements, and widening the **intercostal** space. It seems something is wrong here.

医生:双侧乳房对称,皮肤正常,心尖搏动正常,心前区无异常隆起。但是,您的右侧胸廓饱满,呼吸运动减弱,肋间隙增宽。看来这里有问题了。

Mr. Li: Is it serious?

李先生:严重吗?

Doctor: Take it easy. I will use **percussion** to check the dullness border of your heart. There is

tympanitic note in your right upper lung. The **cardiac dullness border** is normal.

医生：别紧张，让我再来做一下叩诊。您的右上肺呈鼓音。心脏浊音界正常。

Doctor: I will use the stethoscope to check again. The respiratory murmur in the right side is weakening, while that on the left is normal. The heart rate is regular, and no murmur is heard in the auscultatory valve areas.

医生：我再用听诊器检查一下。右侧的呼吸音减弱，左侧呼吸音正常。心率规整，各瓣膜听诊区未闻及杂音。

Mr. Li: What do the results mean?

李先生：这些结果说明什么？

Doctor: Perhaps there is something wrong with your right lung. But don't worry; I still need to check other body parts to make the final diagnosis.

医生：您的右肺可能有点儿问题。别紧张，我接着给您检查身体其他部位，最后才能诊断。

Doctor: Please curl up your legs, and I will check your abdomen.

医生：请您蜷起双腿，我需要检查您的腹部。

Doctor: Good! The skin is normal. And there is no **subcutaneous varicose vein** in your **abdominal walls**, as well as no **gastrointestinal type** or **peristaltic wave**.

医生：很好，皮肤正常，没有腹壁静脉曲张，没有胃肠型或蠕动波。

Doctor: I will use the stethoscope to check you one more time. Well, no vascular murmur. The **bowel sound** is four times per minute, which is normal.

医生：我再用听诊器检查一下。嗯，没有血管杂音，肠鸣音每分钟 4 次，很正常。

Doctor: Please relax your abdomen. I will take percussion. If you feel **aching**, just tell me.

医生：放松腹部，我做一下叩诊检查。如果有疼痛的感觉，请告诉我。

Mr. Li: I'm feeling OK.

李先生：没感觉疼痛。

Doctor: Good. The liver dullness border is normal, and there is no **shifting dullness**.

医生：好的。肝脏浊音界正常，没有移动性浊音。

Doctor: Relax again. I will perform the **abdominal palpation**. If you feel any aching or discomfort, just tell me.

医生：继续放松，我做一下腹部触诊检查。如果疼痛或者不适，请告诉我。

Mr. Li: I'm OK.

李先生：没有不适。

Doctor: I will use a cotton swab to lightly tickle your body to check whether your **abdominal reflexes** are normal or not. Please cooperate with me.

医生：我需要用棉棒在您的身体上划几下，检查您的腹壁反射是否正常，请您配合一下。

Mr. Li: No problem.

李先生：没问题。

Doctor: It's normal. Then I will check your **externalia**.

医生：一切正常。接下来，我检查一下您的外生殖器。

Doctor: Quite normal, thank you for your cooperation. Now, I will check your limbs to see how your **motor function**, **muscle strength**, and nerve reflexes are. Please follow my instruction.

医生：很正常，谢谢您的配合。现在，我再来检查一下您的四肢，看一下您的运动功能、肌力以及神经系统反射情况。您只需按照我的要求做就可以了。

Mr. Li: OK. We may begin now.

李先生：可以，开始吧。

Doctor: Good. It seems that the functions of your limbs and nervous system are also normal.

医生：很好。看来您的四肢和神经系统的功能也是正常的。

Mr. Li: But doctor, I still feel pain in the right side of my chest, difficulty breathing and I'm breaking into a cold sweat.

李先生：可是医生，我还是感觉右侧胸痛、呼吸困难、直出冷汗。

Doctor: I see. From your general physical examination, I think something is wrong with your lungs. But take it easy, I will offer specific treatment for you. And you will be all right soon.

医生：我知道了。通过全身的体格检查，我判断您的肺脏出现了问题。但是，请不要紧张，我会对您进行有针对性的治疗。您很快就会好起来的。

Mr. Li: OK, thank you so much.

李先生：好的，非常感谢！

Doctor: You are welcome. Take a good rest.

医生：不客气，好好休息。

Part Three   Words and Phrases

第三部分   单词和短语

pneumothorax [ˌnjuːmə(ʊ)ˈθɔːræks] *n.* 气胸

【例句】Lung problems that can affect athletes are asthma, pneumonia and pneumothorax. 足以影响运动员的肺部问题有哮喘、肺炎和气胸。

thorax [ˈθɔːræks] *n.* 胸；胸腔

【例句】The engineers ultimately decided to attach two of the spiral beams to each beetle's thorax. 工程师们最终决定把两个螺旋束放置在每个甲虫的胸腔内。

palpitation [ˌpælpəˈteʃən] *n.* 心悸

【例句】Caffeine can cause palpitations and headaches.

sensation [sen'seɪʃ(ə)n] *n.* 感觉

【例句】Floating can be a very pleasant sensation. 咖啡因能引起心悸和头痛。

lymph [lɪmf] *n.* 淋巴

【例句】When breast cancers did occur they tended to be larger tumors spreading to lymph nodes. 如果乳腺癌的确存在，它们往往是较大的肿瘤，会蔓延到淋巴结。

thyroid ['θaɪrɒɪd] *n.* 甲状腺

【例句】If absorbed through contaminated food, especially milk and milk products, it will accumulate in the thyroid and cause cancer. 如果通过污染食物，特别是牛奶和奶制品吸收，它会积聚在甲状腺上并引起癌症。

trachea ['trekɪə] *n.* 气管

【例句】Once the cells were thriving, the artificial trachea was implanted into the patient. 一旦细胞大量繁殖，人造气管就会被移植到病人体内。

stethoscope ['stɛθəskop] *n.* 听诊器

vascular ['væskjələ˞] *adj.* 血管的

【例句】Research suggests that all such vascular conditions are linked by one common symptom-high blood viscosity. 调查显示，所有的血管疾病都与一个普遍的症状有关，即高血黏度。

murmur ['mɝmɚ] *n.* 低语；低语声

bilateral [ˌbaɪ'lætərəl] *adj.* 双边的

【例句】China and the United States concluded a bilateral trade agreement after long negotiations. 中美两国通过长期谈判后订立了一项双边贸易协定。

symmetric [sɪ'mɛtrɪk] *adj.* 对称的；匀称的

【例句】Writing is symmetric with reading, with all its corresponding fragilities. 写是和读对称的，它具有所有相应的脆弱性。

cardiac ['kardɪæk] *adj.* 心脏的

【例句】The man was suffering from cardiac weakness. 这位男士有心脏衰弱的问题。

anomalous [ə'namələs] *adj.* 异常的；不规则的

【例句】For years this anomalous behaviour has baffled scientists. 多年以来，这个异常的行为一直让科学家们感到困惑。

upheaval [ʌp'hɪvl] *n.* 隆起

precordium [pri:'kɔ:dɪəm] *n.* 心前区，心窝

【例句】The pain may also be felt beneath the precordium. 疼痛也可能出现在胸前区下方。

intercostal [ˌɪntɚ'kastl] *adj.* 肋间的

percussion [pɚ'kʌʃən] *n.* 叩诊

aching ['eɪkɪŋ] *adj.* 疼痛的

【例句】My aching back was the least of my problems. 背部疼痛是我最小的问题。

shifting dullness　移动性浊音

abdominal [æbˈdɑmənl] *adj.* 腹部的

【例句】Excessive amounts of abdominal fat increases your risk for high blood sugar and other health problems. 腹部脂肪过多会增加患上高血糖和其他健康问题的风险。

palpation [pælˈpeʃn] *n.* 触诊

【例句】In palpation, a doctor feels the shape and firmness of tissue. 在触诊中,医生能够感受到组织的外形及硬度。

abdominal reflex　腹壁反射

externalia [ekstəːˈneɪlɪə] *n.* 外生殖器

Phrases and Expressions

tympanitic note　鼓音

cardiac dullness border　心脏浊音界

subcutaneous varicose vein　静脉曲张

abdominal walls　腹壁

gastrointestinal type　胃肠型

peristaltic wave　蠕动波

bowel sound　肠鸣音

motor function　运动功能

muscle strength　肌力

accompanied with　伴有,兼有

complain of　主诉,抱怨

fix one's gaze on　注视

body parts　身体部位

curl up　蜷起

cotton swab　棉棒

follow one's instruction　按照……的要求做

（陈　战　刘晓杰）

第四章
心电图

Part One   Case Presentation

Mr. Zhang, a 55-year-old male, is hospitalized with **retrosternal** crushing chest pain accompanied by **nausea** and **vomiting** for the past two hours, and is diagnosed with acute myocardial infarction (AMI). He complains of experiencing sudden retrosternal crushing chest pain radiating to his left shoulder and back when he was climbing stairs two hours ago. He broke into a cold sweat and felt sick. The symptoms remain even after taking a rest. Soon afterwards he vomited once, regurgitating the complete contents of his stomach. He took a pill of **sublingual** nitroglycerin, but ten minutes later experienced no relief. Then he dialed 120 to the **emergency** center to be hospitalized and receive emergency treatment. In order to have a better knowledge about his condition and to make a correct diagnosis, the doctor is going to do an **electrocardiograph** (ECG) for him. The following is their conversation.

第一部分   病 案 介 绍

张先生,55 岁,因胸骨后压榨性疼痛,伴恶心、呕吐 2 小时入院,诊断为急性心肌梗死。病人主诉其于 2 小时前爬楼梯,突然感觉胸骨后压榨性疼痛,向左肩、背部放射,出冷汗,很恶心,休息后未缓解。随后呕吐一次,为胃内容物。舌下含服硝酸甘油一片,10 分钟后无缓解。随后拨打 120 急诊入院。为了更好地了解病人情况,明确诊断,医生需要给病人做心电图检查,以下是他们的对话。

Part Two   Dialogue

第二部分   对   话

Doctor: Hello, Mr. Zhang. I'm the doctor in charge of your case. In order to have a better knowledge about your condition and to make correct diagnosis, I will do an ECG examination for you. It will take about five minutes, OK?

医生：您好！张大爷，我是您的主管医生，为了了解您的身体状况，明确诊断，我需要给您做一次心电图检查。大约需要 5 分钟的时间，可以吗？

Mr. Zhang: OK. But what is an ECG examination?

张先生：好的。但是什么是心电图检查？

Doctor: ECG is a technology that takes a **graphical** recording of the cardiac cycle produced by an electrocardiograph from your body's surface. It reflects the process of signals of excitement transmitting in the heart and the functional condition of the heart. It is one of the important ways to diagnose heart diseases.

医生：心电图是利用心电图机从体表记录心脏每一心动周期所产生的电活动变化图形的技术。它能反映出兴奋在心脏内传播的过程及心脏的功能状态，是目前诊断心脏病的重要方法之一。

Mr. Zhang: That's good. I will cooperate with you.

张先生：好的，我会配合的。

Doctor: Thank you. There is no pain in an ECG examination, so please take it easy. Please put aside your mobile phone and wrist watch to avoid any **interference** to the electrical signals. Then take off your footwear, and unbutton your jacket to expose your chest.

医生：谢谢！心电图检查没有什么痛苦，您完全不用紧张。请您解除手机、手表等物品，防止干扰。然后脱去鞋袜，解开上衣，充分暴露前胸。

Mr. Zhang: I'm ready. May we begin?

张先生：准备好了，可以开始了吗？

Doctor: Yes. Please relax your body and breathe smoothly. I will **smear** some **ethyl alcohol** in your body to help display the **waveform** more clearly. Don't be nervous.

医生：可以了。请您放松身体，平静呼吸。我需要在您的身体上涂一些普通酒精，以便清晰地显示波形，请您不要紧张。

Mr. Zhang: OK, I will try to relax.

张先生：好的，我会放松的。

Doctor: Good! Then I will put the ECG **leads** on your body. Please don't speak, and breathe smoothly.

医生：很好！接下来，我要在您的身体上安放导联。请不要讲话，平静呼吸。

Doctor: It is beginning the tracing, and it will be completed soon.

医生：开始描记图形，很快就好。

(Five minutes later ...)

（5分钟后……）

Doctor: Your ECG is completed, so I will remove the leads. Please wipe your body and get dressed. Thank you for your cooperation.

医生：心电图做好了，我给您撤去导联。您可以擦干身体，穿好衣服了。感谢您的配合！

Mr. Zhang: What about my ECG result?

张先生：我的心电图结果怎么样？

Doctor: Your ECG results are as follows: leads V1-V5: ST-segment **elevation**; QRS complexes displaying Qr type; T wave **inversion**. These show that the **antetheca** of your heart is in the state of infarction.

医生：您的心电图结果显示，V1-V5导联：ST段向上抬高；QRS波群呈Qr型；T波倒置。这些都显示，您心脏的前壁出现梗死。

Doctor: But don't be nervous. We will make a comprehensive therapeutic schedule for you based on your conditions and the results of other **auxiliary** examinations.

医生：不过，请您不要紧张，我们会结合您的身体情况和其他辅助检查的结果，给您制订综合的治疗方案。

Mr. Zhang: OK, I will definitely cooperate with your treatment. Thank you!

张先生：好的，我一定积极配合治疗。谢谢！

Doctor: Good. Here is your call bell. If you feel uncomfortable or need anything, please ring the bell. I will come back right away.

医生：很好，这里有一个呼叫铃。如果有什么不舒服或者其他需要，您可以随时按铃。我会马上过来。

Mr. Zhang: This has been quite helpful, thank you very much!

张先生：这个很有帮助，非常感谢您！

Doctor: You are welcome. Please take a good rest.

医生：不客气，请好好休息。

Part Three　Words and Phrases

第三部分　单词和短语

retrosternal [retroʊˈstɜːnəl] *adj.* 胸骨后的

nausea [ˈnɔːziə] *n.* 恶心

【例句】I was overcome with a feeling of nausea. 我有一种恶心的感觉。

vomit [ˈvɑmɪt] *n. v.* 呕吐

【例句】She began to vomit blood a few days before she died. 她在去世前几天开始吐血。

sublingual [sʌbˈlɪŋgwəl] *adj.* 舌下的；舌下腺的

【例句】With the right sublingual medicine for genital herpes, you can stop herpes outbreaks from recurring. 只要用对了舌下药物，疱疹就不会再次发作了。

emergency [ɪˈmɜˈdʒənsi] *n.* 紧急情况；突发事件

【例句】They were held together to deal with emergency. 他们团结一致以应付紧急情况。

electrocardiograph (ECG) [ɪˌlektroʊˈkɑːdɪɡrɑːf] *n.* 心电图

【例句】An ECG was done before the exercise and immediately after. 分别在运动之前和之后做了心电图。

graphical [ˈgræfɪkl] *adj.* 图解的；绘画的

【例句】A graphical representation of results is shown in figure 1. 图 1 中显示了图解表示的结果。

interference [ˌɪntɚˈfɪrəns] *n.* 干扰，冲突

【例句】Airlines will be able to set cheap fares without further interference from the government. 如果不受政府更多的干预，各航空公司将能够把票价定得很低。

smear [smɪr] *v.* 涂抹

【例句】My sister smeared herself with suntan oil and slept by the swimming pool. 我妹妹用防晒油涂抹了全身，然后睡在那游泳池边。

waveform [ˈweɪvfɔːrm] *n.* [物][电子] 波形

lead 导联

elevation [ˌɛlɪˈveʃən] *n.* 提高

inversion [ɪnˈvɜˈʃən] *n.* 倒置；反向

antetheca [ˌænti'θiːkə] *n.* 前壁

auxiliary [ɔːgˈzɪlɪəri] *adj.* 辅助的；附加的

【例句】The government's first concern was to augment the army and auxiliary forces. 政府首

要关注的是扩充军队与后备军。

Phrases and Expressions

ethyl alcohol　　酒精

break into　　突然开始

functional condition　　功能状态

put aside　　把……放在一边

get dressed　　穿好衣服

as follows　　如下

base on　　基于,以……为根据

（陈　战　刘晓杰）

第五章
晨间护理

Part One   Case Presentation

Mrs.Liu is 60-year-old，who has been admitted to the **Intensive Care Unit (ICU)**, for an infective exacerbation of her **chronic obstructive pulmonary disease (COPD)**. She has been a heavy smoker for approximately thirty years and has not been able to cut down her habit at all. Her medical history also includes **deep vein thrombosis (DVT)** and depression. At present she becomes short of breath at the slightest level of exertion and is very weak, listless, and depressed; she is dependent on a low flow oxygen device.

第一部分   病案介绍

刘女士，60岁，因慢性阻塞性肺部疾病感染性恶化被收入重症监护室。她有近30年严重吸烟史，从未减轻。病史还包括深静脉血栓和抑郁。此刻，她在轻微用力后变得更加气短，也很虚弱、情绪低落并抑郁，依赖于低流量氧疗。

Part Two   Dialogue

第二部分   对   话

Nurse: Good morning Mrs. Liu, my name is Wang Fang; I'm your charge nurse. You can call me Xiao Wang.

护士：早上好，刘阿姨，我叫王芳。我是您的责任护士，您可以叫我小王。

Mrs. Liu: Hi, Xiao Wang.

刘女士: 嗨,小王。

Nurse: How do you feel today?

护士: 今天感觉怎么样?

Mrs. Liu: Oh, just so-so.

刘女士: 噢,还行吧。

Nurse: Would you like some help to wash up?

护士: 你需要帮助清洗吗?

Nurse: I can help you wash up now, if you are ready?

护士: 如果你准备好了,我现在可以帮你清洗。

Mrs. Liu: All right.

刘女士: 好的。

Nurse: I'll just get your wash-clothe, soap, toothbrush, and toothpaste from your drawer ... Let's brush your teeth first, OK?

护士: 我把你的洗脸毛巾,香皂,牙刷,牙膏从你的抽屉里拿出来…我们先刷牙,好吗?

Mrs. Liu: OK. But I'm afraid I can't get up.

刘女士: 好的,但我恐怕起不来。

Nurse: Don't worry. You needn't get up. I will use cotton ball to clean your teeth.

护士: 没关系,你不用起来,我用棉球给你清洁牙齿。

Mrs. Liu: All right.

刘女士: 好吧。

Nurse: (Use forceps to pick up a moistened cotton ball) This is a cotton ball saturated with saline solution. I will use it to clean your teeth. Now, open your mouth, please.

护士: (用镊子夹取一个湿棉球)这是生理盐水棉球,我将用它来给你清洁牙齿。现在,请把嘴巴张开。

Mrs. Liu: OK. (Open mouth)

刘女士: 好的(张开嘴巴)。

Nurse: (Clean the patient's teeth from inside to outside. Use one cotton ball every time.) OK, your teeth are all clean. Can you rinse the mouth by yourself?

护士: (由内向外依次擦洗病人的牙齿。一次只用一个棉球)好了,每个牙齿都擦过了。你能自己漱口吗?

Mrs. Liu: Um, I'm not sure. Can I try?

刘女士: 嗯,很难说。让我试试。

Nurse: Of course. Here's a straw. Try to use it to rinse your mouth and spit into the emesis basin.

护士: 当然可以。这是一根吸管,试着用它来帮你漱口,把脏水吐在弯盘内。

Mrs. Liu: OK. (Rinse the mouth)

刘女士：好的（漱口）。

Nurse: Now, let me help you to clean your face. Is the water temperature OK, or is it too hot or too cold?

护士：现在我来帮您洗脸。水温好吗？太烫或太凉吗？

Mrs. Liu: It's OK.

刘女士：水温正好。

Nurse: (Immerse washcloth in water and wring thoroughly. Fold washcloth around fingers to form a mitt.) First, I'll wash your eyes. Please close your eyes ... Right ... Would you like to use soap on your face?

护士：现在我帮你洗脸（将毛巾浸湿并拧干，缠绕在手上形成手套）。首先，先洗眼睛，请把眼睛闭上…… 对……你要用肥皂洗脸吗？

Mrs. Liu: No, thanks.

刘女士：不用，谢谢。

Nurse: OK. Now, let me wash your forehead，cheeks, nose, neck, and ears.

护士：好，现在洗前额、双颊、鼻子、颈部和耳朵。

Mrs. Liu: My hair must be so disheveled. Is it?

刘女士：我的头发肯定很蓬乱吧？

Nurse: Yes. But you needn't worry. I will tidy it up for you.

护士：是的。不过别担心，我会帮你梳理的。

Mrs. Liu: That's wonderful.

刘女士：太好了。

Nurse: (Comb hair for the patient.) Now, you feel better, don't you?

护士：（给病人梳头）你现在好点了吗？

Mrs. Liu: Yes. Thank you very much.

刘女士：是的，感觉好多了。谢谢。

Nurse: It's my pleasure. You may rest now. Do you mind my opening the windows to air the room a little?

护士：不用谢。你现在可以休息了。你介意我打开窗户通通风吗？

Mrs. Liu: Sure.

刘女士：当然不介意。

Nurse: I'll come back to close them for you later.

护士：稍后我会回来帮您关上窗户的。

Mrs. Liu: Thanks.

刘女士：多谢。

Nurse: Goodbye.

护士：再见。

Mrs. Liu: Goodbye.

刘女士：再见。

Part Three Words and Phrases

第三部分　单词和短语

Intensive Care Unit (ICU)　重症监护室

【例句】Emergency Medicine of the process is divided into the first-aid "Pre-hospitalemergency, Emergency disposal, ICU observation" three stages. 急救医学把急救的过程分为"院前急救、急诊处置、ICU 观察"三个阶段。

exacerbation [ɪɡ,zæsə'beʃən] *n.* 恶化

【例句】For several days, he has had an exacerbation of ulcer symptoms. 几天来，他的溃疡症状加重了。

chronic obstructive pulmonary disease (COPD)　慢性阻塞性肺部疾病

【例句】Chronic obstructive pulmonary disease (COPD) is a common lung disease. 慢性阻塞性肺疾病（COPD）是一种常见的肺部疾病。

approximately [ə'prɔksimətli] *adv.* 大约

【例句】The plane will be taking off in approximately five minutes. 飞机大约五分钟后起飞。

thrombosis [θrɔm'bəusis] *n.* [病理] 血栓形成；血栓症

【例句】Thrombosis is the formation of a blood clot in a person's heart or in one of their blood vessels, which can cause death. 血栓是指在人的心脏或血管里血凝块的形成，可以导致死亡。

deep vein thrombosis (DVT)　深静脉血栓形成

【例句】DVT can be detected through medical testing and can be treated. 深静脉血栓形成可通过医学检测发现并可予以治疗。

depression [di'preʃ(ə)n] *n.* 沮丧；抑郁症

【例句】Depression is an illness like heart disease or cancer. 抑郁是种病，就像是心脏病或癌症一样。

exertion [iɡ'zə:ʃn] *n.* 发挥；努力；劳累

【例句】Nothing lay ahead of us but exertion, struggle, and perseverance. 在我们的脑海里，只剩下了努力，奋斗，锲而不舍。

listless ['lis(t)lis] *adj.* 倦怠的；无精打采的

【例句】They say the children remain feverish, listless and without appetite. 他们说孩子们仍然发热，无精打采，没有胃口。

depressed [di'prest] *adj.* 沮丧的；萧条的；抑郁的

【例句】I feel much depressed. 我感到很沮丧。

Phrases and Expressions

cut down　削减；减少

short of breath　呼吸短促

saturated with ...　浸透……

spit into ...　吐出到……

immerse ... in water　把……浸到水里

wring thoroughly　彻底绞干

fold ... around fingers　把……缠绕在手上

be disheveled　蓬乱，凌乱

（孙瑞丽）

第六章
皮肤护理

Part One　Case Presentation

Mrs. Sun, a 60-year-old female, is admitted because of **progressive swelling** for 3 days and is **diagnosed** with **renal insufficiency**. Because she has a history of heart disease and was exhibiting a fast heartbeat, shortness of breath, and high blood pressure caused by acute left heart failure, she has been transferred to intensive care unit. **Noninvasive ventilator** assisted **ventilation** was begun, and she has also had a central **venous catheter** inserted. Continuous renal replacement **therapy** (CRRT) treatment was given. Now her vital signs have become stable.

第一部分　病 案 介 绍

孙女士,60岁,因全身渐进性浮肿3天入院,诊断为肾功能不全,既往心功能不全病史,因心跳快,呼吸促,血压高,考虑患者急性左心衰发作转入ICU,予无创呼吸机辅助通气,并予紧急右股静脉留置血透管,予患者持续行床边CRRT治疗,患者生命体征逐渐平稳。

Part Two　Dialogue

第二部分　对　　话

Nurse A: Mrs. Sun, how are you feeling now?

护士 A: 孙阿姨,您好! 现在感觉怎么样?

Mrs. Sun: Much better than before.

孙女士: 比之前好多了。

Nurse A: You've been lying in bed like this about 2 hours, let's help you to turn.

护士 A: 您这样平躺了有差不多两小时了,我们帮您转转身吧?

Mrs. Sun: I don't really want to turn, I'm really tired at the moment, would you mind coming later to do this treatment?

孙女士: 我太累了,不想动,你可以晚点再来吗?

Nurse A: Don't worry Mrs. Sun. We will keep an eye on this tube for you. Your edema is really serious, so if you don't move for few hours, your skin can be easily broken, especially in your sacrum area.

护士 A: 您放心,我们会帮您看着这条管的,您身体水肿得很厉害,长时间不动局部皮肤受压容易压坏的,尤其骶尾部。

Nurse B: And we have two nurses here to help. You don't need to move yourself at all.

护士 B: 而且我们两个人帮您,不用您自己用力的。

Mrs. Sun: Okay then.

孙女士: 那好吧。

Nurse A: Which side do you prefer to lie on?

护士 A: 你现在想转向哪边休息?

Mrs. Sun: Right side, please.

孙女士: 右边。

Nurse A: OK. We will help you lie down first, and move up a little bit. Put your hands in front of your **chest** instead of the edge of your bed, bend your left knee and keep your right leg flat because of the **central** venous catheter. Now we are going to turn.

护士 A: 好的。我们先帮您放低点床头,整个人睡向床头一点。手不要抓着床栏,双手可以放在肚子上。右大腿有血透管要放平,左膝盖弯曲,准备翻身了。

Nurse B: Let me check the skin of your back side. Your **sacrum** area and heels are really red.

护士 B: 我现在检查一下您后面的皮肤,您这骶尾部和脚跟都有点压红了。

Mrs. Sun: Will that be all right?

孙女士: 应该没什么大问题吧?

Nurse B: It should be all right after we use some skin protection products, which are useful for redness in areas that receive pressure. I put a pillow behind your back, so you can lie on one side for a while and give the other side a break, also I put a pillow under your left leg. Please do not bend your right leg.

护士 B: 暂时没有,我们给您用点保护皮肤的药,对受压变红的皮肤很有帮助。我给您背后面放一个枕头您这样侧着睡一会儿,让另一侧休息一下。左腿下面也放一个。右腿尽量不要弯曲了。

Mrs. Sun: Okay.

孙女士：好的。

Nurse B: Do you feel comfortable like this?

护士 B: 这样睡得舒服吗？

Mrs. Sun: Yes, I'm comfortable at the moment, but later, when I'm tired, can I remove this pillow and turn myself?

孙女士：可以。我如果累了可以自己把枕头拿掉并转身吗？

Nurse A: You have a central venous catheter in your right leg for CRRT treatment, and your heart still hasn't recovered very well. So before we remove this catheter, it is better that we help you turn. When you are tired, you can call for help anytime.

护士 A: 您现在右大腿有中央静脉根管在做持续血透，而且心脏还没恢复。因此在拔管前，最好我们协助您转身。如果您累了，可以随时叫我们帮忙。

Nurse B: And we will come to see you often, in order to providing the best skin care. When your situation becomes more stable, we will show you how to do bed exercise.

护士 B: 而且，我们也会经常过来帮您的，并帮助您保护皮肤。等您情况稳定点了，再教您在床上活动身体。

Mrs. Sun: That's very nice of you to do that. Thank you very much!

孙女士：你们真是太好了。谢谢你们。

Part Three   Words and Phrases

第三部分   单词和短语

progressive [prə'grɛsɪv] *adj.* 进步的；先进的 *n.* 改革论者；进步分子

【例句】The progressive future belongs to them, because they are already living it. 进步的未来属于他们，因为他们已经生活在其中。

swelling ['swɛlɪŋ] *n.* 肿胀；膨胀；增大；涨水 *adj.* 膨胀的；肿大的；突起的 *v.* 肿胀；膨胀；增多；趾高气扬（swell 的 ing 形式）

【例句】The swelling on her leg was dispersed by cold compresses. 冷敷消除了她腿上的肿块。

diagnose [ˌdaɪəg'nos] *vt.* 诊断；断定 *vi.* 诊断；判断

diagnosed *v.* 诊断；被诊断为（diagnose 的过去分词）

【例句】The doctor diagnosed the illness as pneumonia. 医生诊断这病为肺炎。

renal ['rinl] *adj.* [解剖] 肾脏的，[解剖] 肾的 *n.*（Renal）人名；（法）勒纳尔

【例句】They must be monitored in the long term to ensure that their renal function will not be impaired. 必须对这些小孩进行长期监测才能确定他们的肾脏功能是否受到损伤。

insufficiency [ˌɪnsəˈfɪʃənsi] *n.* 不足, 不充分; 功能不全; 不适当

【例句】Fear arises out of this inner insufficiency, poverty and emptiness. 恐惧来源于这种内在的不足, 贫乏和空虚。

noninvasive [ˌnɒnɪnˈveɪsɪv] *adj.* 非侵袭的; 非侵害的

【例句】But analyzing the gases coming off the old books is noninvasive. 然而, 分析气体的技术实现了非侵入性研究古书。

ventilator [ˈvɛntɪletɚ] *n.* 通风设备; 换气扇; 【医】呼吸机

【例句】The ventilator inventor's adventure prevented him from venturing revenge. 通风机发明家的奇遇阻止了他冒险复仇。

ventilation [ˌvɛntlˈeʃən] *n.* 通风设备; 空气流通

【例句】If humidity not within the set point, turn on external ventilation.
如果湿度不在设置点内, 那么打开外部通风。

venous [ˈvinəs] *adj.* 静脉的; 有脉纹的

【例句】Minor cuts usually produce what is known as venous bleeding. 小伤口通常会引起静脉出血。

catheter [ˈkæθɪtɚ] *n.* [医] 导管; 导尿管; 尿液管

【例句】He expects that his catheter will cost about the same as those used currently. 他希望他的发明能与现在正在普遍使用的导尿管价格一样。

therapy [ˈθɛrəpi] *n.* 治疗, 疗法

【例句】Some patients in therapy want to learn to find satisfaction in what they do. 有些治疗中的病人想学习在他们所做的事情中找到乐趣。

sacrum [ˈsekrəm] *n.* [解剖] 骶骨; [解剖] 荐骨

【例句】It's important to feel comfortable so use blankets or cushions under your head, back or sacrum. 舒适放松是很重要的, 所以在你的头部, 背部和骶骨处放些毯子和垫子。

chest [tʃɛst] *n.* 胸, 胸部; 衣柜; 箱子; 金库

【例句】She snuggled up to his chest. 她偎依在他的胸前。

central [ˈsɛntrəl] *adj.* 中心的; 主要的; 中枢的 *n.* 电话总机

【例句】In all this discussion, moreover, we have so far omitted a central consideration. 另外, 在所有这些讨论中, 到目前为止, 我们忽略了一个主要的考虑。

（胡亚南　王芳芳）

第七章
抹身更衣

Part One   Case Presentation

Mrs. Zhang, a 55-year-old female, has been hospitalized with "abdominal pain for the past two days, which become more serious in the last half day". Examinations showed intestinal **necrosis**, so she had surgery immediately during the night. After the surgery she had two **pelvic drainage** tubes and her blood pressure was low, so she has been admitted into the intensive care unit for better monitoring. The second day after the surgery, Mrs. Zhang is fully awake, but looked tired. Her vital signs were stable. In the afternoon, nurses are going to give a bed bath to her.

第一部分   病案介绍

张女士,55 岁,因为"腹痛 2 天,加重半天"入院,检查考虑肠坏死,半夜立即行了手术治疗。术后留置两条盆腔引流管,术后血压偏低,转入重症医学科监护治疗。术后第二天,患者已经清醒,精神疲倦,生命体征暂时平稳。准备予患者行床上擦浴更衣。

Part Two   Dialogue

第二部分   对   话

Nurse: Mrs. Zhang, how are you and how is your abdominal pain now?

护士:张阿姨,您怎么样了,肚子还痛吗?

Mrs. Zhang: It's much better now.

张女士：好多了。

Nurse: You just had surgery yesterday, and you can't take a shower yourself, so I and another nurse assistant will help you with a bed bath, and change your clothes, is that OK with you?

护士：您昨天刚做完手术，暂时还不能下床洗澡，等下我和护工就给您在床上擦一下身子，再换一套干净的衣服，可以吗？

Mrs. Zhang: That's great, I've been sweating a little.

张女士：太好了。刚好我有点儿出汗了。

Nurse: OK, I will switch off the air condition first, the water temperature is around 45℃. Would you like to check if it is OK for you?

护士：好的。空调我暂时先关了，水温刚量过差不多45℃，我给您在手上试一下看这样的水温合适吗？

Mrs. Zhang: Mm, the temperature is good.

张女士：恩，这个温度可以。

Nurse: Okay, later if you feel cold or uncomfortable, please let us know anytime.

护士：好的，等下如果觉得水温偏凉或者身体觉得冷或其他不舒服可以随时跟我们讲。

Mrs. Zhang: Okay. Thank you.

张女士：好的。谢谢。

Nurse: We will help you lie down first. I'm going to wash your face now. (2 minutes later) Now I need to remove your **sleeve** nearest to me, and wash your arm. (2 minutes later) Now please turn left, so I can wash your back. Don't worry, we will watch your tubes, and keep them in position. Nurse assistant will help you with the other side. And now we'll change your clothes. (5 minutes later)

护士：我们先帮您躺下。现在帮您洗一下脸。（2分钟后）现在帮您脱下我这边的袖子，给您擦下这边胳膊。（2分钟后）现在请转向左边，我帮您擦下背。不用担心身上的各种管道，我们会帮您整理固定好的。护工会给您擦另一边。现在给您换上干净衣服。（5分钟后）

Nurse: Because you have a **urine** catheter, and we need to wash your urine catheter too, in order to protect you from infection.

护士：您现在留置尿管，为预防感染，尿管也要给您冲洗清洁一下。

Mrs. Zhang: That's OK, thank you.

张女士：好的，谢谢你们。

Nurse: Do you feel any discomfort?

张女士：有感觉不舒服吗？

Mrs. Zhang: No, you are doing very well. Don't worry, I will let you know if I'm uncomfortable.

张女士：没有。你们放心做吧，不舒服我会说的。

Nurse: Okay, now we need to get a fresh basin of water, and **soak** your hands and feet.

护士：好的，现在我们换一下水，等会再泡一下手和脚。

Mrs. Zhang: I feel much more comfortable now, after the wash. Thank you very much.

张女士：擦洗了一下我感觉舒服多了，谢谢你们。

Nurse: You are welcome, we're just doing our job. Later when you are able to get out of bed, we can assist you to shower in the bathroom. I have also fixed those two **tubes** in position, so don't worry, but you still need to pay attention to them.

护士：别客气，这都是我们应该做的。等您好一点儿了不用待在床上的时候，我们就可以协助您洗澡，术口这两条引流管，我已经给您固定好了，一般不会牵扯到，但还是要稍微注意一下。

Mrs. Zhang: Okay, it's very nice of you to do this. Thank you.

张女士：好的。太感谢你们了！

Part Three　Words and Phrases

第三部分　单词和短语

necrosis [nɛˈkrosɪs] *n.* 坏死；坏疽；骨疽

【例句】Is there any area of necrosis? 有任何坏死的区域吗？

pelvic [ˈpɛlvɪk] *adj.* 骨盆的

【例句】However, detailed analysis of pelvic bones and teeth confirmed the mummy is a boy despite its female adornments. 然而，尽管有那些女性装饰品，但骨盆骨和牙齿的详细分析证实木乃伊是个男孩。

drainage [ˈdrenɪdʒ] *n.* 排水；排水系统；污水；排水面积

【例句】Pour some gravel into the bottom of your pot for drainage. 倒些沙砾在你地里的底部以用来排水。

sleeve [sliv] *n.* [机]套筒，套管；袖子，[服装]袖套 *vt.* 给……装袖子；给……装套筒

【例句】He pulled my sleeve, attracted my attention in this way. 他扯了扯我的衣袖以引起我的注意。

urine [ˈjʊrən] *n.* 尿

【例句】It goes out of us through urine, through sweat, and even through exhaling. 我们的身体通过排尿、出汗，甚至是呼吸将水排出体外。

soak [soʊk] *vt.* 吸收，吸入；沉浸在（工作或学习中）；使……上下湿透 *vi.* 浸泡；渗透 *n.* 浸；湿透；大雨

【例句】Let it soak for a few hours in warm water. 把它在热水中浸泡几小时。

tube [tuːb] *n.* 管；电子管；隧道；电视机 *vt.* 使成管状；把…装管；用管输送 *vi.* 乘地铁；不及格

【例句】Heat the glass tube to the point that it can bend. 将玻璃管加热，以能弯曲为度。

（胡亚南　王芳芳）

Chapter Eight   Oral Care for Patient with ETT

第八章
气管插管病人的口腔护理

Part One   Case Presentation

Mrs. Zeng, a 40-year-old female, has been hospitalized with **hemorrhage** necrosis **pancreatitis**. She had surgery and was transferred into intensive care unit after the surgery. She needs mechanical ventilation. Mode: SIMV+PS, tidal volume 400ml, respiration rate: 16 times/min. PEEP: 8cmHg, PS: 12cmHg, FIO_2: 60%. Blood gas showed: PH: 7.360, PO_2: 92mmHg, PCO_2: 33.3mmHg, BE: −6mmol/L, AB: 24mmol/L. Hb: 73g/L, Ca^{2+}: 1.8mmol/L. Blood pressure was 78/48 mmHg.

第一部分   病 案 介 绍

曾女士,40 岁,因反复腹痛被诊断为出血坏死性胰腺炎,行手术治疗,术后予转重症监护室。转入后予经口气管插管接呼吸机辅助通气,模式:SIMV+PS, TV 400ml, f 16 次 / 分, PEEP 8cmHg, PS 12cmHg, FIO_2 60%。查血气 PH 7.360, PO_2 92mmHg, PCO_2 33.3mmHg, BE−6mmol/L, AB 24mmol/L。Hb 73g/L, Ca^{2+} 1.8mmol/L。血压 78/48 mmHg,予对症处理。

Part Two   Dialogue

第二部分   对   话

Nurse 1: Morning, Mrs. Zeng. I'm Wang Fang in charge of you today. Can you hear me? If you can, please nod your head.

护士 1: 早上好曾女士,我是您今天的主管护士王芳。您听到我说话就轻点一下头,好吗?

Nurse 1: You still have a tube inside your mouth, so you can't talk at the moment. After your doctor removes this tube, you will be able to talk. Now if you need anything, you can use this pen and paper, or nod your head.

护士 1: 您现在口腔里还有一个气管插管，暂时说不了话，等您好转了医生会给您拔管，然后就能说话了。现在有什么需要帮忙的可以用纸笔和我们简单沟通，或者轻轻点头摇头。

Mrs. Zeng writes: This tube is very uncomfortable, can you remove it now?

曾女士写字： 口里的管太不舒服了，现在能拔掉吗？

Nurse 1: Mrs. Zhang, I understand you feel discomfort. But we can't remove this tube right now and you should never pull it out by yourself. It's very dangerous, okay?

护士 1: 曾女士我知道您不舒服，但现在还不能拔出，您千万不要自己拔出来了。那样会有危险，知道吗？

Mrs. Zeng: (Nod head)

曾女士：（点头）

Nurse 1: Now I'm going to help with your **oral** care. Because of this tube, I need to use the special toothbrush to make it more clean, and reduce the risk of infection. This is Nurse Liu Dan, she and I will both help you with oral **hygiene**. Please cooperate with our instructions.

护士 1: 我们现在帮您清洁一下口腔，您口里有这根管，要用专用的牙刷，这样清洁更彻底，而且可减少口腔内细菌感染风险。这位是刘丹护士，她将和我一起为您做清洁。等会请您根据我们指示配合一下。

Mrs. Zeng: (Nod head)

曾女士：（点头）

Nurse 1: Now we will do your **sputum suction** first, it may cause some discomfort.

护士 1: 现在先帮您吸痰清除下气道口鼻腔分泌物，会有点儿不适。

Nurse 1: Lean your head towards me, please. And Xiao Liu, please release the fixed line, and hold the tube with your hand to keep it in the right side.

护士 1: 头偏向我这一侧。小刘，松开气管插管固定带，手固定好气管插管并将其保持在右侧。

Nurse 2: It is released. The scale is 24cm.

护士 2: 已经松开，刻度 24 厘米。

Nurse 1: Mrs. Zeng, please open your mouth a little bit, I need to remove the **bite-block** first, please be careful not to bite the tube. It's similar to brushing your teeth. Don't worry, the water I flushed into your mouth won't be able to go down to your lungs, it will be sucked away immediately.

Nurse 1: 曾女士，请把嘴巴张大一点儿，我取出右边牙垫，牙齿不要闭合咬到管。如同刷牙一样，冲洗口腔的水不会进入你的肺，马上会吸走，不用担心。

Nurse 2: Mrs. Zeng, we finished the left side. Now I'm going to brush the right side of your mouth.

护士 2: 曾女士,我们已经洗完了左边,现在要清洗管的右侧边的口腔。

Nurse 1: OK, the right side is clean too. Now I only need to put in a bite-block beside the tube inside your mouth, then it's done.

Nurse 1: 好了,右边也清洁完了。再放一个牙垫在您口腔偏左边固定就好了。

Nurse 2: The scale is still 24cm.

护士 2: 刻度还是 24 厘米。

Nurse 1: OK, are you feeling better now, Mrs. Zeng?

护士 1: 好的,曾女士现在口里感觉舒服点儿吗?

Mrs. Zeng: Nod head.

曾女士: 点头。

Nurse 1: Is there anything else I can do for you?

护士 1: 还有别的需要帮助的吗?

Mrs. Zeng: (Shake head)

曾女士:(摇头)

Nurse 1: OK, if you need anything just ring the bell.

护士 1: 好的。有任何需要随时按铃。

Part Three　Words and Phrases

第三部分　单词和短语

pancreatitis [ˌpænkrɪəˈtaɪtɪs] *n.* [内科] 胰腺炎

【例句】The elevated triglycerides seem to interfere with the circulation of the pancreas and cause severe inflammation, known as pancreatitis. 高水平的甘油三酯似乎干扰胰腺的循环,造成严重的炎症,即众所周知的胰腺炎。

tidal volumn *n.* 潮气肺容物

oral [ˈɔrəl] *adj.* 口头的,口述的 *n.* 口试;(Oral) 人名;(土) 奥拉尔

【例句】He lucked out on the oral examination. 他侥幸通过了口语考试。

hygiene [ˈhaɪdʒin] *n.* 卫生;卫生学;保健法

【例句】Many diseases proceed from negligence of hygiene. 许多疾病源于不讲卫生。

sputum [ˈspjʊtəm] *n.* [生理] 痰;唾液

【例句】Is there any blood in your sputum? 你的痰液里有血吗?

suction [ˈsʌkʃən] *n.* 吸;吸力;抽吸

【例句】They use their ample lips to suction out the meat. 它们用自己丰满的嘴唇吸出其中的肉。

bite-block   *n.* 牙垫

（胡亚南   王芳芳）

第九章

服药指导

Part One　Case Presentation

Mr. Zhang, a 70-year-old male, has been hospitalized with acute **pulmonary** infection of chronic **bronchitis** and **right heart failure**. His temperature is 38.9℃ and he had shortness of breath at the time of admission. His charge nurse will give treatments such as cooling in accordance with the doctor's advice. Nurse will guide him on how to take his medication and below is their conversation.

第一部分　病 案 介 绍

张先生,70 岁,因"慢性支气管炎急性发作合并肺部感染,右心衰竭"入院。入院时体温 38.9℃,呼吸急促,遵医嘱给予降温等治疗。管床护士将要给予病人正确的服药指导,以下是他们的对话。

Part Two　Dialogue

第二部分　对　　话

Nurse: Hello, Mr. Zhang. I have some new medicine that the doctor has prescribed for you. You have to start taking them today.

护士:您好,张先生。医生开了一些药物,今天就要开始服用。

Mr. Zhang: Oh, what for?

张先生：哦，这些药物是要做什么用的？

Nurse: This is a medicine for your heart. It will improve your heart function.

护士：这是治疗你心脏的药物。它能够改善心脏功能。

Mr. Zhang: I see. How often do I take it?

张先生：我明白了。这种药片怎么服用？

Nurse: Please take one tablet once a day, after breakfast time.

护士：每次 1 片，每天 1 次，早饭后服用。

Nurse: You have been coughing for a long time, here is some cough syrup.

护士：你咳嗽很长一段时间了，这是止咳糖浆。

Mr. Zhang: How do I take the syrup?

张先生：这种糖浆怎么服用？

Nurse: One teaspoonful, three times a day. Do not drink water right after taking the syrup.

护士：每天 3 次，每次一勺。服药后不宜立即饮水。

Nurse: Your body temperature is 38.9℃ now, this medicine can help lower your body temperature.

护士：你的体温达到了 38.9℃，它能帮助你降低体温。

Mr. Zhang: Then how do I take these tablets?

张先生：这种药怎么服用？

Nurse: When your body temperature is over 38.5℃, take the medicine no more than three times a day, and each time take one tablet. Also, drink more water to promote sweating.

护士：当你体温超过 38.5℃服用，每天不超过 3 次，每次 1 片。同时，请多喝水，促进排汗。

Mr. Zhang: Thank you very much.

张先生：非常感谢你！

Nurse: You are welcome.

护士：不客气。

Part Three   Words and Phrases

第三部分   单词和短语

pulmonary ['pʌlmənɛri] *adj.* 肺的；有肺的；肺状的

【例句】All patients had pulmonary thromboembolism. 所有的病人都有肺血栓栓塞。

failure ['feljə] *n.* 失败；故障；失败者；破产

【例句】Acute heart failure is a clinical syndrome. 急性心力衰竭是一种临床综合征。

tablet ['tæblɪt] *n.* 药片，小片

【例句】Dissolve the tablet in warm water. 把药片放进温水中溶化。

syrup ['sɪrəp] *n.* 含药糖浆，果汁

【例句】Mother dosed the child up with cough syrup. 母亲让孩子按量服用止咳糖浆。

teaspoonful ['tispʊnˌfʊl] *n.* 一茶匙的量

【例句】The other medicine is for his cough. Give him one teaspoonful three times a day. 另一种是止咳药水，每次一茶匙，一天三次。

bronchitis [brɒŋ'kaɪtɪs] *n.* [内科] 支气管炎

right heart failure 　右心衰竭

Phrases and Expressions

in accordance with　　依照；与……一致

shortness of breath　　气促；呼吸浅短

（袁　娟）

第十章
留置胃管

Part One　Case Presentation

Mr. Zhang, a 54-year-old male, hospitalized with right lower **abdominal** pain lasting 12 hours was diagnosed with acute **suppurative appendicitis**. The patient felt abdominal pain which began in the region of the **umbilicus** with associated nausea, and vomiting beginning 12 hours ago. Then the pain localized into the right lower quadrant where the tenderness increased in intensity. Emergency appendectomy was performed on the patient. The patient's vital signs were stable but he had nausea and abdominal distention after surgery. The charge nurse will insert an NG tube for the patient following the doctor's orders, and below is their conversation.

第一部分　病案介绍

张先生，54 岁，因 "右下腹急性疼痛" 12 小时入院，诊断为急性化脓性阑尾炎。病人 12 小时前出现脐周痛，同时伴有恶心及呕吐。后疼痛固定于右下腹并出现疼痛加剧。入院后急诊行阑尾切除术。术后病人生命体征平稳，但出现恶心、呕吐、腹胀。责任护士遵医嘱要给病人插胃管，以下是她们的对话。

Part Two　Dialogue

第二部分　对　　话

（*The patient has just **vomited** a second time, a large amount of **stomach** liquid. He is one day **post-op**.*）

（病人术后第一天，刚才已经是第二次呕吐，吐出大量胃内容物。）

Mr. Zhang: I feel very sick to my stomach, I'm going to throw up again. Where is my **emesis** basin?

张先生：我感觉胃里特别不舒服，又要吐了，我的盂盆呢？

Nurse: Here it is. I need to insert an **NG** tube to help stop your vomiting.

护士：盂盆在这里。为缓解呕吐，我要给您插个胃管。

Mr. Zhang: What is an NG tube?

张先生：什么叫胃管？

Nurse: It is a tube going from your nose to your stomach.

护士：胃管就是从鼻子插到胃里的一根管子。

Mr. Zhang: Will it hurt?

张先生：插胃管会痛吗？

Nurse: It may be uncomfortable going in, but it will empty your stomach. It will go in easily if you follow my instructions.

护士：插的过程中会有不舒服，但是通过胃管可以把胃里的东西排出来。插的过程中如果您配合就会比较容易。

Mr. Zhang: I'll try.

张先生：好吧，我尽力吧。

Nurse: Okay, bend your head so your chin touches your chest. Now I am going to put this tube in your nose. Have you ever had a broken nose or nose surgery?

护士：好，低头让下颌靠近胸部。我要把这个管子通过鼻子插进去，您的鼻子有受伤或做过手术吗？

Mr. Zhang: No.

张先生：没有。

Nurse: Take a sip of water through this straw. **Swallow** a little more. Now raise your head and keep swallowing. Okay, I need to check the placement.

护士：用吸管喝口水，咽下去。现在抬起头，做吞咽动作。好，让我检查一下是否插到胃里了。

(*Nurse uses a stethoscope and* **syringe** *to* **auscultate** *the placement in the stomach.*)

（护士用一个听诊器和注射器检查胃管是否在胃里。）

Nurse: It's in your stomach. I need to tape it to your nose. Thank you. It's working now. This should help relieve your vomiting.

护士：插进去了，现在我要把这个管子固定在您鼻子上。好，胃管已经插好了，您的恶心可以得到缓解了。

Mr. Zhang: How long will the tube be in?

张先生: 这个管子需要留多长时间啊?

Nurse: It depends on how you are feeling. Usually not too long. You can ask the doctor when he comes to examine you this afternoon. This tube may make your throat sore. We can order a throat-spray or mouth rinse if necessary.

护士: 得看您的恢复情况,一般不会太长。今天下午医生来检查时您可以咨询一下他。这个管子可能会使您的咽喉部疼痛,严重时可以用点喷剂或漱口液。

Mr. Zhang: Thank you very much.

张先生: 非常感谢。

Nurse: You are welcome, see you soon.

护士: 不客气,我一会会来看您的。

Part Three　Words and Phrases

第三部分　单词和短语

suppurative ['sʌpjuəretɪv] *adj.* 化脓的;化脓性的;使化脓的

【例句】The cerebrospinal fluid assumes the suppurative change.
脑脊液检查提示化脓性改变。

appendicitis [ə,pɛndə'saɪtɪs] *n.* [医] 阑尾炎;盲肠炎

【例句】Appendicitis is one of the most common surgical problems.
阑尾炎是最常见的外科疾病之一。

umbilicus [ʌm'bɪlɪkəs] *n.* 脐,种脐;中心

stomach ['stʌmək] *n.* 胃;腹部;胃口

【例句】Every time after I run, I feel sick in my stomach and my teeth. 每次跑完步,我感觉从口腔到胃都非常难受。

emesis ['ɛməsɪs] *n.* [临床] 呕吐

【例句】Nothing is given by mouth, and the patient's head is turned to one side to avoid aspiration if emesis occurs. 为防止呕吐时发生误吸,病人要禁食水,头偏向一侧。

swallow ['swalo] *vi.* 吞下;咽下

【例句】Polly took a bite of the apple, chewed, and swallowed. 波莉咬了一口苹果,咀嚼后咽了下去。

syringe [sɪ'rɪndʒ] *n.* 注射器;洗涤器

【例句】She grabs a syringe from her tray and stabs him in the arm. 她从托盘里拿出一个注射器刺入他的手臂上。

auscultate [ˈɔskəlˌtet] *vi.* 听诊

【例句】The students were taught how to auscultate chest with stethoscope. 教学生用听诊器听诊胸部。

Phrases and Expressions

post-op *adj.* ［口语］=postoperative　手术后

NG tube = nasal gastric tube　鼻胃管

NPO［拉丁语］(=nothing by mouth)　禁饮食

（潘兰霞）

Chapter Eleven   Gastrointestinal Nutrition (Nasogastric)

第十一章
胃肠内营养（鼻饲）

Part one   Case Presentation

Mrs. Feng, a 55-year-old female, has been hospitalized with "**dizziness**, nausea, and **vomiting** for half day after a fall". Her head CT scan shows cerebral infarction. The patient has a weak right side leg and arm and she has difficulty swallowing. In order to ensure she gets sufficient nutrition and avoids **aspiration**, her doctor ordered feeding tube intubation. Below is the **dialogue** between patient and nurse.

第一部分   病 案 介 绍

冯女士,55 岁,因为"跌倒后一过性意识丧失,伴头晕,恶心呕心半天"而入院,头颅 CT 提示脑梗死。患者右侧肢体乏力,吞咽困难,为保证患者营养及避免患者误吸,予患者留置胃管鼻饲饮食。

Part Two   Dialogue

第二部分   对　　话

Nurse: Mrs. Feng, how are you feeling today? Your lunch is here, are you hungry?

护士:冯女士,您好! 您的午餐送过来了,肚子饿了没?

Mrs. Feng: Yes, a little bit.

冯女士:有点儿饿了。

45

Nurse: Do you want to eat now?

护士：那现在吃点儿？

Mrs. Feng: OK.

冯女士：好的。

Nurse: We will feed you through this feeding tube to your stomach.

护士：等下还是要从鼻子里的这根胃管打到胃里去。

Mrs. Feng: OK, when can I start eating by myself?

冯女士：哦，好的。那我什么时候可以自己吃？

Nurse: We will assess your ability to swallow, and when you are able to eat by yourself, we will remove this feeding tube. Before this, your function **rehabilitation therapist** will help you.

护士：这个要等您的吞咽功能完全恢复了，才可以自己吃。康复专家会帮助您做吞咽方面的锻炼，评估您何时适合吃什么样的食物。

Mrs. Feng: Okay.

冯女士：好的。

Nurse: Let me check the temperature of the food first.

护士：我先量下食物的温度。

Mrs. Feng: I normally don't eat cool food.

冯女士：我平时不喜欢吃太凉的。

Nurse: OK, but maybe you don't want too hot, either, now it is around 41℃, which is just fine.

护士：好的。不过也不要吃太热的哦。现在 41℃，刚好适合。

Mrs. Feng: OK.

冯女士：好的。

Nurse: I will raise the head of your bed now, and help you sit up a little bit. Also I need to check your feeding tube to see if it is still in position.

护士：那我先要摇高床头，坐起来点再吃。现在检查一下您的胃管是不是还在胃内。

Mrs. Feng: I have been getting hungry very easily lately, can you feed me more, please?

冯女士：我这两天感觉饿的好快，可不可以每次多打点？

Nurse: Yes, a little bit more, but maybe not too much at one time, in case you feel nausea after we lower the head of your bed. However, when you feel hungry, you just ring the bell and we will feed you more, OK?

护士：可以稍微多一点，不过不要一次吃得太多了，怕你到时候反流误吸就不好了。您感觉到饿了的时候就给我们说一下，我们评估您胃内的已经消化了就再给你吃，好吗？

Mrs. Feng: OK, thank you .

冯女士：好的，谢谢。

Nurse: You had 350ml just now, do you feel full?

护士：吃了 350ml, 饱了吗？

Mrs. Feng: Yes, I feel full now.

冯女士：恩，饱了。

Nurse: OK, we will let you lie like this for a half hour, then we will help you lie down, okay?

护士：好的，那您这样坐着休息半小时，然后我们会帮助您躺下，好吗？

Mrs. Feng: OK, you go and do your work. When I'm ready, I will ring the bell.

护士：好的。你先去忙吧，想躺下去的时候我会按铃。

Nurse: OK, I will see you later then.

冯女士：知道了。一会儿见。

Part Three　Words and Phrases

第三部分　单词和短语

dizziness ['dɪzənɪs] *n.* 头晕；头昏眼花

【例句】Doctors have been left baffled by her condition which causes dizziness and can trigger a seizure. 这种病发作起来会头昏眼花，并可能引发癫痫，这难倒了许多医生。

vomiting ['vɑmɪtɪŋ] *v.* 呕吐（vomit 的 ing 形式）

【例句】Never prepare food for others if you have diarrhea or vomiting. 如果你腹泻或呕吐，千万不要为他人准备食物。

aspiration [ˌæspəˈreʃən] *n.* 渴望；抱负；送气；吸气；吸引术

【例句】He nurses an aspiration to be a poet. 他心怀当诗人的愿望。

dialogue ['daɪəˌlɔg] *n.* 对话；意见交换 *vi.* 对话 *vt.* 用对话表达

【例句】The dialogue remained light and friendly. 对话仍然是轻松友好的。

rehabilitation [ˌriːəˌbɪlɪˈteʃn] *n.* 复原

【例句】They also benefit less from prevention efforts, and have less access to high-quality treatment and rehabilitation services. 他们也较少能受益于预防工作，而且较少能获取高质量的治疗和康复服务。

therapist ['θɛrəpɪst] *n.* 临床医学家；治疗学家

【例句】I returned to my therapist, Jake, to discuss the incident. 我回到我的治疗师杰克那里讨论这件事。

（胡亚南　王芳芳）

Chapter Tweleve　Blood Sugar (Glucose) Monitoring

第十二章
血糖监测

Part One　Case Presentation

Mrs. Li is 55 years old. Because she had been eating a lot of greasy food the past three days, she presented persistent **colic**, accompanied with **abdominal distention** and nausea. After being admitted into the emergency department and having an examination, she was diagnosed with **severe pancreatitis**. She followed treatments of **fasting**, **gastrointestinal decompression**, **pancreatic juice** and gastric acid secretion inhibition, and symptomatic treatment as ordered by her doctor. Now her **stomachache** and abdominal distention are **alleviated** but her blood sugar levels continue to be high, so she has been transferred to the intensive care unit (ICU). The patient now has an **insulin pump** to regulate blood sugar levels. In order to adjust insulin dosage, her charge nurse is going to monitor her **blood sugar**, and below is their conversation.

第一部分　病 案 介 绍

李女士，55 岁，三日前因进食大量油腻食物后，出现上腹部疼痛，呈持续性绞痛，伴发腹胀、恶心，送入医院的急诊科进行相关检查，确诊为重症胰腺炎。遵医嘱给予禁饮食，胃肠减压，抑制胰液，抑酸，对症治疗后，腹痛、腹胀有所减轻，但血糖值一直偏高，为进一步诊治转入重症监护室。目前，病人用胰岛素持续泵入以调节血糖水平。为了调整病人胰岛素的用量，管床护士将要对病人进行血糖监测，以下是她们的对话。

Part Two   Dialogue

第二部分   对   话

Nurse: Hello, Mrs. Li, I'm your charge nurse, Meng Li. You can call me Xiao Meng. I need to use a **glucose meter** to monitor your blood sugar, it will take about 2 minutes, is that OK?

护士：你好，李女士，我是您的主管护士孟丽，你可以叫我小孟，我需要使用血糖仪来监测您的血糖，大概需要 2 分钟的时间，可以吗？

Mrs. Li: Hello, Xiao Meng, that's OK, but why do I need to monitor blood sugar?

李女士：你好，小孟，可以的。为什么我要监测血糖？

Nurse: Your blood sugar levels have been very high since admission, so we need to monitor it regularly to adjust the insulin dosage.

护士：您这几天的血糖值一直都很高，我们需要定时测一下血糖水平，来调整胰岛素的用量。

Mrs. Li: Okay, but why is my blood sugar so high all the time? I am not a diabetic.

李女士：哦，那我的血糖为什么会一直高呢？ 我之前没有糖尿病。

Nurse: Because your pancreas was inflamed, which destroyed some insulin secretion cells. There is not enough insulin in your body now, so your blood sugar level increased.

护士：因为您的胰腺发炎，破坏了很多分泌胰岛素的细胞。现在您身体里的胰岛素不够，血糖就高了。

Mrs. Li: OK, I see. How do I use this little meter?

李女士：好的，我知道了。这个小仪器怎么用呢？

Nurse: Don't worry. You only need to cooperate with me while I do it for you. Which finger you would like to be pricked? First, I need to disinfect the surface of this finger.

护士：您不用担心。您只需要配合我就可以了。您想扎哪个手指？ 首先我要给这只手指表面消毒。

Nurse: Secondly, I need to prick this finger. It will hurt a little.

护士：然后我需要用针扎一下您的手指，会有点儿疼。

Nurse: Now, we use one drop of blood to test. The result will come out only in 5 seconds.

护士：现在取一滴血进行检测。5 秒钟结果就出来了。

Mrs. Li: How is my blood sugar?

李女士：我的血糖值怎么样？

Nurse: Your blood sugar level is 13.4mmol/L, which is still high.

护士: 您的血糖值是 13.4mmol/L，这次还是有些偏高。

Nurse: Okay, I'm finished. I'll come back in two hours to run the test again. Now, is there anything else I can do for you?

护士: 好了我做完了，我在两个小时以后还会来给您测一下血糖值。现在，还有什么其他需要我可以帮您做的吗？

Mrs. Li: I still have a stomach ache and dry mouth. Could you please give me some water to drink?

李女士: 我还是觉得肚子痛，口干，你可以给我喝点水吗？

Nurse: In your current condition you are not allowed to drink water, but I can wet your lips with moist swab. I will report your stomachache to your doctor, and here is your call light, if you need anything before I come back to see you, please ring the bell.

护士: 您现在的情况还不可以喝水，不过我可以用棉签蘸水给你湿润一下嘴唇。我会把腹痛汇报给您的医生来处理，这里有个呼叫铃，如果在我回来之前您有什么需要的，请随时按铃。

Mrs. Li: Okay, thank you very much.

李女士: 好的，非常感谢你！

Nurse: You are welcome, see you soon.

护士: 不客气，马上回来。

Part Three　Words and Phrases

第三部分　单词和短语

colic ['kɒlɪk] *n.* 绞痛

【例句】But how do you know if they are experiencing colic symptoms?
但你怎么知道他们是否经历着绞痛症状？

abdominal distension　腹胀

severe pancreatitis　重症胰腺炎

【例句】The aim is to explore the treatment method of acute and severe pancreatitis after renal transplantation. 目的为探讨肾移植术后急性重症胰腺炎内科综合治疗的方法和疗效。

fasting ['fɑːstɪŋ] *n.* 禁食

【例句】Following the instructions I was given, I started fasting the day before the procedure. 按照指导，我在手术前一天就开始禁食了。

gastrointestinal decompression　胃肠减压

pancreatic juice   *n.* 胰液

stomachache ['stʌməkeɪk] *n.* 腹痛

【例句】Or maybe during the meal, you are feeling a stomachache. 或者在吃饭的时候,你会感到胃部疼痛。

alleviate [ə'liːvieɪt] *v.* 减轻

【例句】Nowadays, a great deal therapies can be done to alleviate back pain. 现在,有很多可以实施的疗法以减轻背部疼痛。

insulin ['ɪnsjʊlɪn] *n.* 胰岛素

【例句】Check your blood sugar level before and after any activity, especially if you take insulin. 活动前后,尤其是使用了胰岛素,需要监测血糖水平。

pump [pʌmp] *v.* 泵入

【例句】The pump analogizes with the human heart. 水泵被用来比拟人的心脏。

pancreases ['pæŋkrɪəs] *n.* 胰腺

【例句】All the patients accept conventional therapy, including gastrointestinal decompression, to correct water-electrolyte and acid-base balance and parenteral nutrition. 所有的患者都接受常规的治疗,包括胃肠道减压,以纠正水电解质和酸碱平衡和肠道营养。

blood sugar/ blood glucose   血糖值

glucose meter   血糖仪

【例句】A blood-glucose meter is used to detect glucose level in blood.
血糖仪是用于测量血液中葡萄糖含量的仪器。

Further Reading

aggravate ['ægrəveɪt]   *v.* 加重

hypoglycemia [ˌhaɪpəuglaɪ'siːmɪə]   *n.* 低血糖

hyperglycemia [ˌhaɪpəglaɪ'siːmɪə]   *n.* 高血糖

（周　芬）

第十三章

采集静脉血

Part One   Case Presentation

Mrs. Lei is 78-years-old, hospitalized with abdominal pain that was mild for 5 days, and has become serious in the last day. Her body check suggested **acute diffuse peritonitis**, **gastrointestinal perforation**. She had surgery immediately. After the surgery her vital signs are not stable, so, considering her medical history with coronary heart disease and cardiac insufficiency, she has been transferred to intensive care unit for better **monitoring**. Her temperature was 38.5℃, and her heart rate was 120 beats per minute. Her blood pressure was 80/50mmHg, respiration rate was 26 times per minute, and her oxygen saturation was 95%. The second day after treatment, her vital signs became stable. Her doctor prescribed blood sampling and emergency biochemistry, blood lactate and other items.

第一部分　病案介绍

雷女士,78 岁,因腹部疼痛 5 天,加重 1 天而入院。检查提示急性弥漫性腹膜炎,消化道穿孔,紧急行手术治疗。术后考虑患者有冠心病,心功能不全病史,且目前患者病情不稳定,于是转入重症医学科。转入时患者体温 38.5℃,心率 120 次 / 分,血压 80/50mmHg,呼吸 26 次 / 分,血氧饱和度 95%。予对症处理,术后第二天生命体征逐渐平稳。医生开出抽血检查血常规及急诊生化,血乳酸等项目。

Part Two   Dialogue

第二部分   对   话

Nurse: Morning, Mrs. Lei.

护士：雷女士，早上好！

Mrs. Lei: Morning!

雷女士：早！

Nurse: I'm the nurse in charge of your case, how are you feeling today?

护士：我是您的主管护士王芳，今天感觉怎么样？

Mrs. Lei: Much better than yesterday, but I still feel pain in my **abdomen**, and I feel very tired.

雷女士：感觉比昨天好多了，不过肚子还是有点痛，觉得很疲倦。

Nurse: You just had surgery yesterday, it takes time. Don't worry. Now I'd like to take your blood sample for a test, will that be OK?

护士：昨天才做完手术，没这么快恢复，慢慢来，我们一起努力。等下要帮您采集一些血液做检查，可以吗？

Mrs. Lei: Yesterday you took lots of blood, you still want more today?

雷女士：昨天抽过好多血了，今天还要抽吗？

Nurse: Yes, we still need some blood sample for a test today. We need to monitor your **surgical** area to see if it is still bleeding or is infected, and we need to check your electrolyte levels.

护士：恩，是的，今天需要一些血样做测试。因为您昨天做了手术，我们需要监测您的手术部位是否有出血或感染，还要检测您的电解质水平。

Mrs. Lei: I didn't eat anything in the last few days, I don't know if I still have enough blood for you.

雷女士：我这几天都没吃东西，不知道还有没有足够的血。

Nurse: I only need two samples, it's just a very small part of your blood. This is the only way, the doctor will be able to give you a better treatment according to your test results.

护士：我们仅需采集两管血，是您身体的很少的一部分。检测只能使用血液进行。根据检查结果医生能更好地为您治疗。

Mrs. Lei: OK then.

雷女士：嗯，好的。

Nurse: Which arm do you prefer for taking your blood? We normally take from the **elbow**.

护士：那您想抽哪只手呢？我们一般采集肘部血管。

Mrs. Lei: Left side, please.

雷女士：左手吧。

Nurse: OK, let me have a look at your vein first.

护士：好的。我们先检查一下血管。

Nurse: Okay, the left side is all right.

护士：恩，这边血管可以的。

Mrs. Lei: Please be gentle when you take my blood.

雷女士：等下抽血时候轻一点儿。

Nurse: Okay, just relax, it will be over soon. Please **clench** your fist, and do not move your arm.

护士：好的，您放轻松一点儿，很快就会完成的。请先握一下拳头，手臂先不要移动。

Nurse: OK, now you can release your fist. It's finished.

护士：恩，可以松开拳头了，已经采集完了。

Mrs. Lei: OK, thanks.

雷女士：好的，谢谢。

Nurse: Thank you for your co-operation. You go ahead and rest now, and if you need anything, just ring the bell, and I will come to see you as soon as I can.

护士：谢谢您的配合。您先休息，有什么事情随时按铃告诉我，我也会经常来看您的。

Mrs. Lei: That's very nice of you for saying that. See you.

雷女士：好的，谢谢你，再见。

Part Three　Words and Phrases

第三部分　单词和短语

acute [əˈkjut] *adj.* 严重的，[医]急性的；敏锐的；激烈的；尖声的

【例句】A bad tooth can cause acute pain. 一颗蛀牙可以引起激烈的疼痛。

diffuse [dɪˈfjuːz] *adj.* 弥漫的；散开的 *vt.* 扩散；传播；漫射 *vi.* 传播；四散

【例句】The printing press helped diffuse scientific knowledge. 印刷品有助于传播科学知识。

peritonitis [ˌpɛrɪtnˈaɪtɪs] *n.* [内科]腹膜炎

【例句】This will cause nausea, vomiting, abdominal pain, fever, blood in stool, peritonitis (an inflamed, infected lining of the abdomen) and death if not treated quickly enough. 这会引起恶心、

呕吐、腹痛、发热、便血、腹膜炎（一种被感染的腹部内层炎症）以及由于治疗不及时引起的死亡。

gastrointestinal [ˌgæstroɪnˈtɛstɪnl] *adj.* 胃肠的

【例句】Up to half the people who get swine flu never develop a fever, and some suffer from gastrointestinal symptoms as well as more standard flu symptoms. 大约一半的甲流患者都没有发热的症状，许多人除了一般的流感症状外，还会感到胃肠道不适。

perforation [ˌpɝfəˈreʃən] *n.* 穿孔；贯穿

【例句】The 110-decibel level of piling risks perforation of the eardrum, which leads to hearing loss. 打桩作业带来的 110 分贝噪音有可能导致鼓膜穿孔，会导致失聪。

monitoring [ˈmɔnɪtərɪŋ] *n.* 监视，［自］监控；检验，检查 *v.* 监视，［通信］［军］监听，监督（monitor 的 ing 形式）

【例　句】This provides the business with an objective way of monitoring and adjusting its investments. 这为业务提供了一个客观的方法以监控并调整它的投资。

abdomen [ˈæbdəmən] *n.* 腹部；下腹；腹腔

【例句】Scans of his chest, abdomen, and pelvis likewise showed nothing. 扫描他的胸部，腹部和骨盆也没有什么发现。

surgical [ˈsɝdʒɪkl] *adj.* 外科的；手术上的 *n.* 外科手术；外科病房

【例句】In his case a simple surgical operation is indicated. 他的病需要做一个简单的外科手术。

elbow [ˈɛlbo] *n.* 肘部；弯头；扶手 *vt.* 推挤；用手肘推开

【例句】She dug her elbow into his ribs. 她用胳膊肘戳了一下他的肋部。

clench [klɛntʃ] *vt.* 紧握；确定；把……敲弯 *vi.* 握紧；钉牢 *n.* 紧抓；敲环脚 *n.*（Clench）人名;（英）克伦奇

【例句】Don't clench your fists because it can lead to tightness in the arms, shoulders, and neck. 不要紧握你的拳头因为这样会导致你手臂，肩膀和脖子的紧绷。

（胡亚南　王芳芳）

Chapter Fourteen   Inserting/Taking Intravenous Cannulation

第十四章
静脉注射

Part One   Case Presentation

Mr. Wang, 79 years old, has been hospitalized with colon cancer. The patient has been undergoing radical colon cancer treatment and has been in the intensive care unit (ICU) for one day. The clinical symptoms of the patient are pale complexion, local incision pain with general discomfort, and the vital signs and the oxygen saturation of blood are showing 84%. The patient should be treated with an analgesic by venous pump, oxygen therapy with low flow, as well as intravenous treatment. Nurses should make a brief evaluation before the treatment, then offer the venous cannulation so as to administer the different kinds of medication when the patient is in changeable condition, in this regard to keep the patient away from repeated intravenous insertion.

第一部分   病 案 介 绍

王先生, 79 岁, 因结肠癌入院, 全麻结肠癌根治术后住进重症监护病房 1 天。病人面色苍白, 主诉切口疼痛, 周身不适, 生命体征监测血氧饱和度为 84%, 遵医嘱应用止痛泵给药, 持续低流量吸氧, 同时给予静脉输液治疗。治疗前护士需要对病人进行快速评估, 然后再进行静脉留置针穿刺术, 以便随时根据病情持续给药, 从而减少病人需反复多次静脉穿刺的痛苦。

Part Two   Dialogue

第二部分   对   话

Nurse: Good morning, Mr. Wang. I'm your bed nurse Xiao Li, how are you feeling today? Do you still feel pain around your **incision**? I need to give you some medication by the venous **cannulation** according to your symptoms under the doctor's order. It will take about 10 minutes. May I have a look at your hand?

护士：王先生早上好，我是您的管床护士小李，您现在感觉如何？切口处还疼吗？由于您术后病情的需要，遵医嘱我要为您做静脉留置针穿刺，大概需要 10 分钟，我能先看一下您手上的血管吗？

Mr. Wang: Morning Xiao Li (speaking in a very low voice), I am still feeling pain from the incision and some general discomfort, but I can't describe it exactly. That's okay, please go ahead.

王先生：（声音微弱地）你好小李，我的切口处很疼，全身不舒服，也说明白不哪儿难受。好，你先看看吧。

Nurse: I will roll up your sleeve first. Please make a slight fist, is it painful here?

护士：我把袖子先给您挽上。请您轻轻攥拳，我按的地方疼吗？

Mr. Wang: Ah ... It is not too painful.

王先生：呃……还不算太疼。

Nurse: I am going to give you the oxygen therapy, then I will take the venous cannulation for you. Do you need to use the restroom?

护士：好我现在马上给您吸氧，然后就给您打留置针用药，您需要小便吗？

Mr. Wang: (Weakly) That's all right. I don't need to go to the restroom.

王先生：（虚弱地）好吧，我现在不需要小便。

Nurse: Do you feel any oxygen flow through your nose at present?

护士：您现在能感觉到有氧气流通过鼻孔吗？

Mr. Wang: (Nods slightly) Yes.

王先生：（轻轻点头示意）能。

Nurse: Well, then I will regulate the flow of oxygen at a volume of 2 liters per minute. How are you feeling now?

护士：那好，我先把氧气流量为您调到 2 升 / 分。您现在感觉如何？

Mr. Wang: (Nods again) Okay.

王先生：（轻轻点头示意）还好。

Nurse: I am going to insert the venous cannulation under your skin. Please make a fist again and don't be nervous.

护士：我现在要给您进行静脉留置针穿刺。请您再次轻轻攥拳，不要紧张。

Mr. Wang: (Makes a small noise.) Ah ...

王先生：（轻声喊）啊……

Nurse: I am fixing your cannulation and please be careful not to disrupt this part when you move.

护士：我现在给您固定留置针,请您活动的时候注意不要触碰这个部位。

Mr. Wang: Okay. Thank you for your help.

王先生：行,谢谢您的帮助。

Nurse: You are welcome. If you need any help just press the call bell.

护士：不客气,如有需要请按床头呼叫器。

Part Three　Words and Phrases

第三部分　单词和短语

insert [ɪn'sɜ:t] *vt.* 插入；刺入；进针

【例句】I will insert the needle in you skin, please don't be nervous. 我要在您的皮肤处进针了,请不要紧张。

cannulation [ˌkænjʊ'leɪʃn] *n.* 管子中空,套管插入式

【例句】Cannulation taking is very useful for patient's treatment. 插管在治疗患者时非常有用。

oxygen ['ɒksɪdʒən] *n.* 氧气

【例句】We can't live without oxygen. 我们无法离开氧气生存。

Phrases and Expressions

keep ... from　免于……,避免……

different kinds of　不同种类的,各种各样的

（安雪梅）

第十五章
静脉输液

Part One　Case Presentation

Mrs. Song is 60-year-old, who used to be a preschool teacher. She said that she caught a cold after going out into the wet two days ago. She took her temperature with a thermometer at home and her temperature was 39.5℃. She tried to lower her temperature on her own, but there was no improvement before she went to the hospital. The patient presented with a phlegmy cough and shortness of breath. Close observation of the patient's vital signs show a pulse of 110 and blood pressure of 120/74mmHg. Her respiration was at 30 breathes a minute. During further observation the doctor noted bilateral diffuse **crackles** when he used **auscultation**. A subsequent blood gas analysis (ABG) showed pH 7.45, PaO$_2$ 50mmHg. The patient's face was showing **cyanosis** and she gave continuous positive airway pressure oxygen intake. She is to take 1g cefazolin sodium and put it into 100ml **dextrose** 5% in water solution by the doctor's orders. In order to get the cooperation from the patient, the primary nurse needs to assess the condition of patient and explain the aim of intravenous infusion. The primary nurse must review the physician's order before intravenous infusion, including the patient's name, the bed number, age, sex, the condition, the history of allergy, her willingness to cooperate, and ask the patient if she or he needs to urinate or poop. Below is their conversation.

第一部分　病案介绍

宋女士,60 岁,小学教师。主诉:两天前淋雨后感冒,在家中测得体温 39.5℃,经在家中降温效果不明显,后入院治疗。患者表现为咳嗽多痰、气促,生命体征监测脉搏 110 次 / 分,血压 120/74mmHg,呼吸 30 次 / 分,医生听诊患者双侧肺底有湿啰音,血气分析报告显示 pH 为 7.45,氧分压为 50mmHg,病人面色发绀,立刻给予无创呼吸机辅助通气,遵医嘱给 5% 葡萄糖盐水溶液 100ml,加入头孢唑林钠 1g 静脉滴注。为了取得病人配合,责任护士需要评估病人,向病人讲解输液的目的并取得合作;责任护士在输液前核对医嘱,包括病人姓名、床号、年龄、性别、病情、询问有无过敏史、合作情况,询问是否需要解大、小便,做好输液前的准备。以下是她们的对话。

Part Two　Dialogue

第二部分　对　　话

Nurse: Good morning, Mrs. Song. I'm the nurse in charge of you. My name is Mary. It's time to give you intravenous infusion. You can use the bedpans before intravenous infusion and I can help you.

护士:您好,宋女士,我是你的负责护士玛丽。现在该输液了,输液前您可以使用便盆先解小便,我可以帮助您。

Mrs. Song: Excuse me, could you tell me about the use of the intravenous fluids?

宋女士:不好意思,您能告诉我这些液体的作用吗?

Nurse: Sure. The fluids will directly supply a dose of cefazolin sodium to cure disease for rapid effectiveness. Meanwhile, it can correct or prevent fluid and electrolyte disturbances that may have resulted from illness.

护士:当然,输液是给您输入头孢唑林钠以快速获得疗效达到治疗疾病的目的。同时,提供水分和电解质,预防和纠正体液紊乱。

Mrs. Song: Is there a way to test the cefazolin sodium by **intracutaneous** injection?

宋女士:输液的药物头孢唑林钠需要做皮试吗?

Nurse: Yes, it is necessary to prevent **anaphylactic** reaction. Are you allergic to any medicine?

护士:是的,需要做,以防发生过敏反应。您对什么药物过敏吗?

Mrs. Song: No, do I still need a test tomorrow?

宋女士:没有。那明天还需要做皮试吗?

Nurse: If the test is negative, you will not need to test by intracutaneous injection tomorrow. But if the test is positive, you cannot use the medicine and I'll inform your doctor. Please do not worry about it.

护士:今天皮试结果如果是阴性的话,明天就不用做了。皮试结果如果是阳性的话,您就不能使用该药物,我会通知医生处理的,请放心。

Mrs. Song: Would you please make the fluid drip more quickly?

宋女士:可以让液体滴快点儿吗?

Nurse: No. Generally, flow rate is 40 to 60 (gtt/min) for normal adults. Slower flow rate is suitable for the elderly. Fluid volume excess occurs when the client has received too much volume and an overly rapid administration of intravenous solutions, which causes a sudden increase of circulating blood volume and puts an overloaded strain on your heart, which can even result in death. Do not change the infusion rate without a nurse's approval, but the slow flow rate is suitable for you. You can press the bedside bell if you need any help. Thank you for your cooperation.

护士：不可以，通常成人滴速为 40~60 滴 / 分，老年人应该滴慢一点儿。如果滴速过快，短时间内输入过多液体，容易发生循环负荷过重，加重心脏负担，会危及生命安全。这个滴速是适合您的，未经护士允许，请您不要随意调节输液速度。您需要帮助时，可以按床头铃。谢谢您的配合。

Part Three　Words and Phases

第三部分　单词和短语

crackle ['kræk(ə)l] ['krækl] *n.* 裂纹；龟裂；爆裂声 *vt.* 使发爆裂声；使产生碎裂花纹 *vi.* 发劈啪声，发出细碎的爆裂声

【例句】Can they feel the crackle of electricity in the wind? 他们能否感受到风中的电光火石？

auscultation [ˌɔːsk(ə)l'teɪʃ(ə)n] [ˌɔskəl'teʃən] *n.* 听诊

【例句】Another diagnostic method is auscultation and olfaction. 另一种诊断方法是听诊和闻诊。

cyanosis [ˌsaɪə'nəʊsɪs] [ˌsaɪə'nosɪs] *n.* 发绀，青紫

【例句】Signs include difficulty breathing, cyanosis, and exercise intolerance. 症状包括呼吸困难、紫绀和运动不耐受。

dextrose ['dekstrəʊz;-s] ['dɛkstroz] *n.* 葡萄糖

【例句】Ten minutes after the scanning began, participants were given a water solution containing dextrose, a type of sugar. 在扫描开始 10 分钟后，参与者得到了一种含有葡萄糖的水溶液。

intracutaneous [ˌɪntrəkjuː'teɪnjəs] [ˌɪntrəkjʊ'teɪnɪrs] *adj.* 皮内的

【例句】Statistics show that bronchial provocation test is better than intracutaneous test. 统计显示，支气管激发试验优于皮内试验。

anaphylactic [ˌænəfɪ'læktɪk] [ˌænəfɪ'læktɪk] *adj.* 过敏的；[医] 过敏性的；导致过敏的

【例句】Yet be warned, additional bites could once again lead to anaphylactic shock. 但被警告，额外的叮咬可能再次导致过敏性休克。

Phrases and Expressions

blood gas analysis (ABG)　血气分析
Continuous Positive Airway Pressure　无创呼吸机（又称持续气道正压通气）
intravenous infusion　静脉输液
cefazolin sodium　头孢唑林钠
electrolyte disturbances　电解质紊乱
intracutaneous injection　皮内注射

（王　芸）

第十六章

留置尿管

Part One   Case Presentation

Mrs. Zhang, 70 years old, has been hospitalized with right abdominal pain lasting for 5 days. After being diagnosed with obstructive **suppurative cholangitis**, she had surgery. After the surgery, the patient started to have **septic** shock symptoms. Her heart rate went to 120 beats/min, respiration rate was 26 times/min, temperature was 39 ℃ , and blood pressure was 76/50mmHg. In order to have better observation of the patient's **fluid**, her doctor ordered **insertion** of a urine catheter.

第一部分   病 案 介 绍

张女士,70 岁,因 "右腹疼痛 5 天" 入院,诊断为梗阻性化脓性胆管炎,之后行了手术治疗。术后患者出现感染性休克症状,心率 120 次 / 分,呼吸 26 次 / 分,体温 39℃ , 血压 76/50mmHg。为监测患者的尿量,医生开出留置导尿的医嘱。

Part two   Dialogue

第二部分   对   话

Nurse: Mrs. Zhang, are you feeling better today?

护士: 张女士,今天感觉好点儿没有?

Mrs. Zhang: Yes, much better with the abdominal pain, but I still feel tired, and a little bit flustered.

张女士: 肚子痛的好了很多,不过好累,有点心慌。

Nurse: Let me see, do you feel full or do you want pee?

护士: 让我看看,肚子胀吗? 有没有想小便?

Mrs. Zhang: No, I don't want pee now.

张女士: 现在不想小便。

Nurse: Your blood pressure is a little bit low now. Your doctor wants to know how your fluids are doing, so we need to insert a urine catheter in you in order to better observe your fluid output, for example, your urine.

护士: 您现在血压有点低,医生需要知道您小便的情况,我现在给您插一个尿管,将尿液引出来就可以随时观察了。

Mrs. Zhang: I can pee by myself.

张女士: 我自己可以解小便。

Nurse: You just had a surgery, and your heart function isn't good. You need good rest, and you can't **get up to** pee all the time.

护士: 那您也不能每小时都解,而且您刚做完手术,心脏功能也不是很好,要多注意休息,不能反复折腾。

Mrs. Zhang: Must I do this?

张女士: 一定要插?

Nurse: Because of your situation now, I'm afraid that's a "yes", so the doctor can have a better understanding of your situation.

护士: 是的,您现在的情况需要,这样医生才能更好地为您治疗。

Mrs. Zhang: OK, will that hurt?

张女士: 好吧。会痛吗?

Nurse: Yes, it will be a little bit uncomfortable. But it won't take long. Let me close the windows first.

护士: 刚插会有一点儿不舒服。不过很快的。等我先关好门窗。

Mrs. Zhang: OK.

张女士: 好。

Nurse: I will help you to take off one side of your trousers first, please open your legs a little bit and stay still for a while.

护士: 我先帮您把这边裤腿脱下来,腿稍分开,暂时不要动。

Nurse: Now I will **sterilize** the area. (Two minutes later) I'm going to insert the catheter. Relax and take a deep breath. OK, it's sufficiently in position now.

护士: 现在给您消毒。(2分钟后)准备插管了,放松,深呼吸。好了,已经插好了。

Mrs. Zhang: Thank goodness. How long shall I keep it in for?

张女士：这个管要留多久？

Nurse: This depends on your situation and your doctor's decision.

护士：这个要医生根据您的病情来决定的。

Mrs. Zhang: Is it in a stable position?

张女士：那它会不会自己掉出来？

Nurse: Yes, it is inserted well. Don't worry, as long as you don't push it, it won't come out. Is there anything else I can do for you?

护士：不会的，我已经给您固定好了。不要担心，您自己不要牵拉它就好了。还有别的需要帮忙的吗？

Mrs. Zhang: No, thanks.

张女士：没有了。

Part Three　Words and Phrases

第三部分　单词和短语

suppurative ['sʌpjʊəretɪv] *adj.* 化脓的；化脓性的；使化脓的 *n.* 吸脓药；化脓促进剂

【例句】The objective is to investigate the features and diagnosis of the acute suppurative osteomyelitis of infant. 目的是探讨婴幼儿急性化脓性骨髓炎的特点及诊断方法。

cholangitis [ˌkɔlən'dʒaɪtɪs] *n.* 胆道炎，[内科] 胆管炎

【例句】He has a long history of biliary tract, or acute cholangitis history with chills, fever, and jaundice. 他有长期的胆道病史，或伴有寒战发热、黄疸的急性胆管炎史。

septic ['sɛptɪk] *adj.* 败血症的；[医] 脓毒性的；腐败的 *n.* 腐烂物

【例句】Put some anti-septic cream on it. 涂上一些防止败血症的药膏。

fluid ['fluɪd] *adj.* 流动的；流畅的；不固定的 *n.* 流体；液体

【例句】The parting of the waters can be understood through fluid dynamics. 水域被分开是可以用流体动力学来理解的。

insertion [ɪn'sɜːʃən] *n.* 插入；嵌入；插入物

【例句】Sometimes the insertion of one word can change the meaning of a whole sentence. 有时插入一个字可以改变全句的意义。

sterilize ['stɛrəlaɪz] *vt.* 消毒，杀菌；使成不毛；使绝育；使不起作用

【例句】He boiled his syringe and fired his knife to sterilize them. 他把注射器放到水中煮，把刀子放在火上烧来进行消毒。

【例句】It's therefore important that projects provide good documentation and other help so volunteers can get up to speed quickly. 因此，重要的是，项目要提供良好的文档材料和其他帮助，志愿者才能迅速赶上。

Phrases and Expressions

get up to　赶上，追上；达到

（胡亚南　王芳芳）

第十七章
检查告知

Background

Computerized tomography surrounds human body some stratification plane through X tube the scanning, surveys and draws in this stratification plane each spot to absorb X data, then use the computer the high-speed operation and the picture reconstruction principle, obtains this stratification plane the cross section picture.

Digital geometry processing is used to generate a three-dimensional image of the inside of the object from a large series of two-dimensional **radiographic** images taken around a single axis of rotation. Medical imaging is the most common application of X-ray CT. Its cross-sectional images are used for diagnostic and **therapeutic** purposes in various medical disciplines. The rest of this article discusses medical-imaging X-ray CT; industrial applications of X-ray CT are discussed at industrial computed tomography scanning. As X-ray CT is the most common form of CT in medicine and various other contexts, the term computed tomography alone (or CT) is often used to refer to X-ray CT, although other types exist, such as positron emission tomography (PET) and single-photon emission computed tomography (SPECT). Older and less preferred terms that also refer to X-ray CT are computed axial tomography (CAT scan) and computer-aided/assisted tomography. X-ray CT is a form of radiography, although the word "radiography" used alone usually refers, by wide convention, to non-tomographic radiography.

CT is regarded as a moderate-to high-radiation diagnostic technique. The improved resolution of CT has permitted the development of new investigations, which may have advantages; compared to conventional radiography, for example, CT angiography avoids the invasive insertion of a catheter. CT **colonography** (also known as virtual colonoscopy or VC for short) may be as useful as a barium enema for detection of tumors, but may use a lower radiation dose. CT VC is increasingly being used in the UK as a diagnostic test for bowel cancer and can negate the need for a colonoscopy.

CT 是通过 X 射线对人体分层平面进行的计算机断层扫描、测量和绘制,并利用计算机处理、重建图像,得到分层的截面图。

数字几何处理用来生成三维图像,它是由二维图像围绕旋转轴形成。医学影像是 X 线

CT 最常见的应用。它的横断面图像用于各种医学学科的诊断和治疗。本文着重讨论医学成像 X 射线 CT；当然也有 X 射线 CT 工业上有着广泛应用。

因为无论在医学或者其他场合，X 射线 CT 是最常见，因此计算机断层扫描（或 CT）通常指的就是 X 射线 CT。当然 CT 也存在其他类型，如正电子发射断层摄影（PET）和单光子发射计算机断层摄影（SPECT）。旧的非专业的术语中也把 X 射线 CT 称为计算机断层扫描（CAT 扫描）和计算机辅助 / 辅助断层摄影。X 射线 CT 是一种放射学的一种形式，尽管"放射"一词常被广泛地用于非体层摄影。

CT 被认为是一种中高量辐射的诊断技术。提高 CT 的分辨率，可以开展新的研究，这具有非常明显的优势；例如与传统的放射学相比，CT 血管成像避免了导管的侵入性操作。CT 结肠术（也称为虚拟结肠镜检查或简称 VC）可能和钡剂灌肠一样可以用于检测肿瘤，而具有较低的辐射剂量。在英国，CT VC 被越来越多地用于诊断肠癌，从而避免了结肠镜检查的必要。

Part One   Case Presentation

Mark was admitted to the hospital for "five years of coughing". He had been hospitalized with chronic obstructive pulmonary disease, lung infection and respiratory failure for many times before. His cough and sputum become aggravated every time when the cold weather come. He took medicine such as ipratropium bromide and budesonide to control those symptoms at home. Doctor Wang decided to let the nurse take him for a CT scan.

第一部分   病 案 介 绍

麦克因"反复咳嗽咳痰 5 年"入院。既往多次因慢性阻塞性肺疾病、肺部感染、呼吸衰竭住院治疗。每因天气变冷时咳嗽咳痰加重，平时服用异丙托溴铵、布地奈德等药物控制症状。王医生决定让护士带 Mark 行胸部 CT 检查。

Part Two   Dialogue

第二部分   对   话

Nurse: Good morning, Mr. Li. Dr. Wang let me take you to have a CT test.

护士：早上好，李先生。王医生让我送您去做 CT 检查。

Mr. Li: Yes, of cause.

李先生：是的，当然。

Radiologist: Mr. Li, I will take a CT scan for you. This will give image of your lung.

放射科医生：李先生，我将为您做肺部 CT 扫描。这将看到您肺部成像的情况。

Mr. Li: All right. What should I do now? Can I see it?

李先生：好吧。现在我应该做什么？我可以看到它吗？

Radiologist: You will lie down on this table for 20 minutes while the CT scan is being taken. I leave you alone but I will be watching you from that glass window there. Don't be afraid, you are safe here, and it won't hurt.

放射科医生：CT 扫描时，您会躺在这里 20 分钟。您独自一人在这里，但我将从玻璃窗看着你。别害怕，您是安全的，它没有伤害。

Mr. Li: I see. Is this dangerous?

李先生：我明白了。有危险吗？

Radiologist: The only risk of CT scan is radiation, the same risk as all other X-ray tests. Overall, the risks of CT are minimal. But the advantages are **enormous**. The entire region of interest can be scanned very fast, usually in a single breath hold. Short scanning time (less than 30 seconds) avoids inconvenience to very sick and restless patients. Very high quality re-constructions including 3-D images can be made.

放射科医生：CT 扫描的唯一风险是辐射。和其他 X 射线测试同样的风险。总的来说 CT 的风险很小。但优势是巨大的。能够快速地扫描整个区域，通常在一次吸气中就能完成。扫描时间短（小于 30 秒）避免给危重病人造成影响。它能提供非常高质量的 3D 图像。

Mr. Li: OK. Is there any pain?

李先生：好吧。会疼吗？

Radiologist: Take it easy, there is no pain. It can be done in a very short period of time; it's safe and fast.

放射科医生：放轻松，没有痛苦。它可以在很短的时间内完成，安全、快速。

Mr. Li: All right. Thank you.

李先生：好吧。谢谢你！

Nurse: Mr. Li, would you come here please, and change into this hospital gown? The radiologist will take your chest X-ray.

护士：李先生。您可以过来换上医院的衣服吗？放射科医生将为您拍摄胸部 X 光片。

Mr. Li: Should I take off all my clothes even my underwear?

李先生：我应该脱掉我所有的衣服包括我的内衣？

Nurse: Not really, you can keep your underwear on. All your belongings can be kept in the **cabinet**.

护士：不是，您可以保留你的内衣。您所有的物品可以放在阁子里。

Mr. Li: All right, I'm done. What should I do next? I am cold now.

李先生：好吧，我完成了。接下来我应该做什么？我现在有点冷。

Nurse: Now, Mr. Li, you may go into room 1. The radiologist is waiting for you.

护士：现在您可以进入 1 号房间。放射科医生在等您。

Radiologist: Hello, Mr. Li. Do you know what kind of X-ray we are going to do?

放射科医生：您好，李先生。你知道我们要做什么样的 X 线检查吗？

Mr. Li: I think my doctor just ordered chest X-ray for me. Is that right?

李先生：我想我的医生让我做胸部 X 光片。是这样吗？

Radiologist: Right. And now you can step on the pedal, turn around and face me. That's right. Now can you keep close to the stand in front of you?

放射科医生：没错。现在您可以踩踏板，转身面对我。这是正确的。现在您可以贴近机器吗？

Mr. Li: Do you mean to press on the stand in front of me as close as possible?

李先生：你的意思是我尽可能靠近机器面前吗？

Radiologist: Exactly, that's what I want you to do. And now I'm going to shoot. Keep yourself straight and don't move. OK, it's done.

放射科医生：没错，这就是我要您做的。现在我要开始了。保持自己站直，不要动。好的，结束了。

Mr. Li: You have done it. Shall I go now?

李先生：我现在可以走了吗？

Radiologist: Oh, yes, you may dress now. The film will be ready in 30 minutes.

放射科医生：哦，是的，您现在可以穿衣服。30 分钟后出片子。

Mr. Li: Thank you.

李先生：谢谢。

Part Three　Words and Phrases

第三部分　单词和短语

computerized tomography 　*n.* 电脑断层摄影术

radiographic [ˌredɪoˈɡræfɪk] *adj.* 射线照相术的

【例句】By making radiographic images of everyday objects, I've found some surprising answers. 通过对日常物体的放射线影像，使我找到了令人吃惊的解答。

therapeutic [ˌθɛrəˈpjutɪk] *adj.* 治疗的；治疗学的；有益于健康的；*n.* 治疗剂；治疗学家

【例句】They hustled Jeanne to accept their therapeutic plan. 他们强迫珍妮接受他们的治疗方案。

colonography   *n.* 结肠成像术

enormous [ɪˈnɔrməs] *adj.* 庞大的,巨大的;凶暴的,极恶的

【例句】But we can not ignore its enormous vitality for its simplicity! 但我们不能因为它的简单而忽视它巨大的生命力。

cabinet [ˈkæbənət] *n.* 内阁;橱柜;展览艺术品的小陈列室 *adj.* 内阁的;私下的,秘密的

【例句】The Prime Minister presides at meetings of the Cabinet. 首相主持内阁会议。

Phrases and Expressions

be regarded as   被认为是
have a CT test   CT 检查
take off   脱掉

（毛　帅）

Chapter Eighteen   Central Venous Catheterization

第十八章
深静脉 /PICC 置管

Background

Central venous catheterization provides for the administration of caustic and critical medications as well as allowing sampling of blood and measurement of central venous pressure. Recent evidence and Institute for Healthcare Improvement bundled guidelines suggest that the **subclavian vein** is the preferred choice for placement of a central venous catheter.

General contraindications for placement of a central venous catheter include infection of the area overlying the target vein and **thrombosis** of the target vein. Specific contraindications to the subclavian approach include fracture of the **ipsilateral** clavicle or anterior **proximal** ribs, which can distort the anatomy and make placement difficult. Greater caution should be used when placing a central venous catheter in **coagulopathic** patients. The location of the artery (beneath the clavicle) makes application of direct pressure nearly impossible in attempts to control bleeding.

中心静脉导管为输注重要药物、反复采样血样和中心静脉压测压提供了方便。最近的证据和医疗指南建议的首选是锁骨下中央静脉导管置管。

一般中心静脉导管置管的禁忌证包括感染和静脉血栓。锁骨下中心静脉导管置管的特殊禁忌证包括同侧锁骨骨折或近端前肋骨骨折,两者会造成解剖变形和置管困难。为凝血功能异常的病人放置中心静脉导管时应更谨慎。另外,由于锁骨下动脉的解剖位置,误穿后试图压迫止血几乎是不可能的。

Part One   Case Presentation

Nurse plans to insert a PICC tube for the patient who need to receive chemotherapy, here she visits Dr. Lee to ask about it.

第一部分　病 案 介 绍

护士计划给接受化疗的病人留置 PICC 管,她向李医生询问了相关的事项。

Part Two　Dialogue

第二部分　对　　话

Nurse: Good morning, Doctor Li. I heard that you can use central line for some people who are going to have chemotherapy that would normally require a lot of injection and blood tests.

护士: 早上好,李医生。我听说您可以为将要进行化疗的患者使用中央静脉导管,这些患者通常需要大量的静脉注射和血液检查。

Dr. Li: Yes, this is PICC. It's used when a people needs intravenous medication chemotherapy, or fluids for an extended period of time.

李医生: 是的,这是 PICC。一般供人们静脉注射化疗药物或需要长时间输入液体时使用。

Nurse: What's about PICC? Can you give me some explanation?

护士: PICC 是什么? 您能解释一下吗?

Dr. Li: Of course. PICC can give a patient repeated or continuous treatments without having to keep finding a vein. The patient can go home with PICC in, and blood samples can be taken from it without having to use a needle each time.

李医生: 当然可以。PICC 可以给病人重复或连续治疗,而不必每次穿刺静脉。病人可以携带 PICC 回家,血液样本也无需每次使用针抽取。

Nurse: Where can I do it? Must be in hospital? And what aftercare will I need to tell the patient?

护士: 在哪里可以做? 必须在医院里吗? 放置后我需要告诉病人什么?

Dr. Li: It isn't easy to look after their own PICC, because they would have to learn to change the dressing and flush the line with one hand! Don't worry if this isn't possible. We will arrange for a district nurse to flush and clean the line for her.

李医生: 患者要照料自己的 PICC 不太容易,因为他们必须学会使用单手脱穿衣物和冲洗! 不要担心。我们将安排一个地区护士帮助患者冲洗和清洁。

Nurse: Is there a risk of the PICC?

护士：PICC 有风险吗?

Dr. Li: Most patients go through their treatment without any problems with their PICC, but there are certain risks involved. But don't worry, we will help them to deal with these problems.

李医生：大多数患者使用 PICC 接受治疗没有任何问题,但是有一定的风险。别担心,我们会帮助他们解决这些问题。

Nurse: Thank you very much. I will come here next week.

护士：非常感谢。我下周会来这儿。

Dr. Li: Goodbye.

李医生：再见。

Nurse: See you later.

护士：再见。

Part Three　Words and Phrases

第三部分　单词和短语

central venous catheterization　*n.* 中央静脉导管置管术

subclavian vein　*n.* 锁骨下静脉

thrombosis [θram'bosɪs] *n.* [病理] 血栓形成;血栓症

【例句】Arms flailed, necks stretched and torsos bent as every passenger attempted to reduce their chances of being hit by deep-vein thrombosis. 捶胳膊,伸脖子,半弯,因为这样可以减少旅客们患深层静脉血栓几率。

ipsilateral [ɪpsɪ'lætərəl] *adj.* 身体的同侧的

【例句】Enlargement of the ipsilateral choroid plexus maybe secondary to hyperplasia orangiomatous involvement. 同侧脉络丛增大,可能是由于过度增生或被血管瘤累及。

proximal ['praksɪməl] *adj.* 最接近的,邻近的;近身体中央的

【例句】Chromosome 5 is distinguished by a proximal knob. 第 5 染色体的特点是有一个近侧的节结。

Phrases and Expressions

attempts to control bleeding   试图控制出血

arrange for   安排

deal with   处理；解决

（毛　帅　张建东）

Chapter Nineteen   Continuous Renal Replacement Therapy

第十九章

肾脏替代治疗

Part One   Case Presentation

Hemodialysis machines are used to replace the renal (kidney) function for people who suffer from end stage renal disease. The function of the dialysis machine is to provide the fluids and other mechanisms necessary for the cleaning of the patient's blood and removal of excess fluid. Operation of these machines must be conducted by trained personnel only. Dialysis machines have multiple alarms that can occur during treatment, and effectively **troubleshooting** these alarms increases dialysis efficiency. In order to accomplish this, it is necessary to approach the management of alarm troubleshooting in a systematic manner.

Dialysis works on the principles of the diffusion of solutes and **ultra filtration** of fluid across a **semi-permeable** membrane. Diffusion is a property of substances in water; substances in water tend to move from an area of high concentration to an area of low concentration. Blood flows by one side of a semi-permeable membrane, and a **dialysate**, or special dialysis fluid, flows by the opposite side. A semipermeable membrane is a thin layer of material that contains holes of various sizes, or pores. Smaller solutes and fluid pass through the membrane, but the membrane blocks the passage of larger substances (for example, red blood cells, large proteins). This replicates the filtering process that takes place in the kidneys, when the blood enters the kidneys and the larger substances are separated from the smaller ones in the **glomerulus.**

第一部分   病 案 介 绍

血液透析机能够替代肾功能应用于终末期肾脏疾病的患者。透析机的功能是利用透析液和其他机制来清洗病人的血液、去除潴留的液体。这些机器必须由受过训练的人员操作。

透析机器在治疗过程中会出现多次警报,有效地排除这些警报可以提高透析效率。为了实现这一目标,需要系统地处理、管理报警故障。

透析的原理包括溶质的扩散和半透膜的超滤。在水中扩散是物质的属性,物质在水中往往从高浓度区域向低浓度的区域运动。血液流动在半透膜的一侧,透析液在另一侧。半透膜是一种薄膜材料,有不同大小的孔。小的溶质和液体能够通过膜,但是大的物质不能(如红细胞、大蛋白质分子等)。这与肾脏的过滤过程相同:血液进入肾脏,肾小球能把分子量较大的物质与较小的物质分开。

Part Two   Dialogue

第二部分   对　话

Intern nurse: Good morning, head nurse.

实习护士:早上好,护士长。

Head nurse: Good morning, girls. Well, first I will introduce the dialysis machine to you.

护士长:早上好,姑娘们。首先,我将给你们介绍透析机器。

Intern nurse: Thank you, head nurse. That will be helpful.

实习护士:谢谢护士长。那太有帮助了。

Head nurse: The dialysis machine has two systems, the **extracorporeal** (outside the body) circuit and dialysate delivery system. The extracorporeal circuit is the tubing, blood pump, heparin (blood thinner) pump, kidney, monitors for blood flow and blood pressure, and air bubbles. The dialysate delivery system of the machine mixes the bath with purified water and checks to be sure it is safe, large to fit through the pores in the membranes, but urea and salt flow through membranes into the sterile solution and are removed.

护士长:透析机器有两个系统,体外(体外)循环和透析液输送系统。体外循环是管道,血泵,肝素泵(血液稀释剂),肾脏,血流量和血压监测器,以及气泡。机器的透析液输送系统将洗涤液和净化水混合,并检查其是否安全并能通过膜的孔隙,并确保尿素和盐通过半透膜进入无菌溶液中并被移除。

Intern nurse: Please introduce the procedure to me.

实习护士:请您介绍下过程。

Head nurse: OK. First, blood from the patient runs through tubes made of a semi-porous membrane. Outside the tube is a sterile solution made up of water, sugars and other components. Then, red and white blood cells and other important blood components are large to fit through the pores in the membranes, but urea and salt flow through membranes into the sterile solution and are removed.

护士长：好的。首先，病人的血液流经半透膜制成的管。管外是由水、糖及其他成分组成的一种无菌溶液。然后，血细胞和白细胞等重要的血液成分大量通过膜的孔隙，但尿素和盐流经膜进入无菌溶液中并被除去。

Intern nurse: Oh, I see. But I don't know what kind of patients will consider hemodialysis?

实习护士：哦，我明白了。但我不知道什么样的病人会考虑血液透析？

Head nurse: When the kidney fails, harmful wastes build up in the body, the blood pressure may rise, and the body may retain excess fluid and not make enough red blood cells. When this happens, you need treatment to replace the work of your failed kidneys.

护士长：肾脏衰竭时，有害废物在体内产生，血压可能升高，身体可能会保留多余的液体，不能制造足够的红细胞。当这一切发生的时候，则需要治疗以替代衰竭的肾脏。

Intern nurse: Where is hemodialysis done? Should it be done at hospital?

实习护士：血液透析在哪里做？必须在医院吗？

Head nurse: Hemodialysis can be done in a hospital, but is usually done in the dialysis center by nurses and trained technicians. It can also be done at home with a help of a partner.

护士长：血液透析在医院可以做，但通常是在透析中心由护士和训练有素的技术人员完成。也可以在家里成员的帮助下完成。

Intern nurse: What is the length of time for dialysis treatments?

实习护士：透析治疗的时间是多久？

Head nurse: Dialysis is done three times a week for 3 to 5 hours. The schedule is very rigid and usually runs on a Monday/Wednesday/Friday schedule or Tuesday/Thursday/Saturday schedule. You have the option to choose a morning, afternoon, or evening shift depending on the availability of the dialysis unit.

护士长：透析每周做三次，每次 3~5 小时。时间表非常严格，通常在周一、周三和周五或周二、周四和周六的时间表上安排。你可以根据透析室的空余时间选择上午、下午或者晚上。

Intern nurse: During dialysis, what will we do with the patient?

实习护士：透析期间，我们能做些什么？

Head nurse: During dialysis, the dialysis staff checks the patient's blood pressure frequently and adjusts the dialysis machine to ensure that the proper amount of fluid is being removed from the patients body.

护士长：在透析期间，透析人员经常检查病人的血压和调整透析机器参数，以确保从病人身体中移除适量的液体。

Intern nurse: OK, thank you.

实习护士：好的，谢谢。

Part Three   Words and Phrases

第三部分   单词和短语

hemodialysis [ˌhɛmədaɪ'ælɪsɪs] *n.*［临床］血液透析；血液渗析

【例句】To cure this disease, there are only two ways: hemodialysis and kidney transplant. 治疗此病只有两种方法：血液透析和换肾。

troubleshooting ['trʌbl ʃuːtɪŋ] *n.* 解决纷争；发现并修理故障 *v.* 检修（troubleshoot 的 ing 形式）；当调解人

【例句】To you and me, that means troubleshooting. 对你我而言，这意味着故障排除。

ultrafiltration [ˌʌltrəfɪl'treʃən] *n.*［化学］超滤，［环境］超滤作用

【例句】Membrane technologies consist of a group of treatment processes which include reverse osmosis, nanofiltration and ultrafiltration. 膜技术由一系列的处理程序组成，其中包含反渗透，纳滤和超滤。

semi-permeable *adj.* 半渗透的

【例句】Pressurized water is passed over a semi-permeable membrane which allows the passage of water molecules while rejecting the passage of larger ions. 受压水经过半渗透膜，使得水分子能通过，而更大的离子却不会通过。

glomerulus [glɔ'merjuləs] *n.*［组织］肾小球

【例句】Each nephron contains a tuft of capillary blood vessels (glomerulus) and tiny tubules that lead to larger collecting tubes. 一个肾单元包含一个毛细血管丛（肾小球）和一个细小的小管（肾小管），进而引导到更粗大的收集管。

dialysate [dai'ælizeit] *n.* 透析液；渗析液

【例句】Extra fluid and waste products are drawn out of your blood and into the dialysate. 超临界流体和废物的产品抽出的血液和透析液进入。

Phrases and Expressions

be used to   习惯于；被用来做

suffer from   忍受；遭受；患……病；受……苦

be conducted by   由……指挥

are separated from   与……分离

made up of   由……组成；由……构成

（毛　帅　张建东）

第二十章
纤维支纤镜吸痰

Part One   Case Presentation

Mr. Gu, a 67-year-old male, is hospitalized because of a cough that has persisted for 10 years, but has become serious in the last 3 days. Considering AECOPD, **antibiotics** were used for infection control, and non-invasive ventilation was used, too. He was coughing yellow and sticky sputum, and at times couldn't sufficiently cough it up. Her lower lungs can hear obvious wet rale. So the doctor ordered **bronchofibroscope** for sputum suction.

第一部分   病 案 介 绍

顾先生,67 岁,因"反复咳嗽 10 余年,气促 8 年,加重 3 天"考虑慢性阻塞性肺病(急性加重期)而入院,入院后予抗生素抗感染,予无创呼吸机辅助通气。患者咳出黄黏痰,有时甚至咳不出,双下肺可以听到明显湿啰音。医生开医嘱准备予患者行纤维支纤镜吸痰。

Part Two   Dialogue

第二部分   对   话

Doctor: Mr. Gu, we checked your lungs and found that there's a lot of sputum inside, and since you have no energy to cough it out, this obstructed your breathing. So I will use a machine to help suck the sputum out. Then you will be able to breathe more smoothly. Also, we will take a sample for a test to find the most suitable medication for you.

医生: 顾先生,您好。我检查了您的肺部,发现肺里面很多痰,但由于自己咳不出来,会阻碍您的呼吸。等会我在机器帮助下将肺里的痰液吸出来,这样气道通畅后呼吸会顺畅一点,而且可以留取痰液做检查是否有感染及何种感染,方便更好地用药。

Mr. Gu: OK, just do what you think is right for me.

顾先生: 好的,听您的安排。

Doctor: OK, you take a rest first. When was the last time you eat?

医生: 那您先休息下,您最后一次吃东西是什么时候?

Mr. Gu: This morning at 7 am I had some porridge, but I didn't have much of an appetite, so I only had a little.

顾先生: 早上 7 点左右吃了点粥,没胃口,后来不舒服就吃了一点儿。

Doctor: It's already been about 4 hours since then, so nurse Wang and I will help you suck the sputum soon.

医生: 那到现在已经有 4 个多小时了,等下我和王护士一起给您做。

Mr. Gu: That's OK.

顾先生: 好的。

Doctor: Nurse Wang, please first give the patient 2% lidocaine **hydrochloride inhalation** for 15 minutes, and get ready for the bronchofibroscope. We start in 15 minutes.

医生: 王护士,先给患者 2% 的利多卡因 100mg 雾化 15 分钟,准备好用物,15 分钟后开始做。

Nurse: OK.

护士: 好的。

(PS: about 15 minutes later)

(约 15 分钟后)

Doctor: Please relax, Mr. Gu, we are going to start now. You just had some medication, so you won't feel much discomfort.

医生: 顾先生,放轻松点,我们现在准备开始了。刚才用了点麻药,应该没那么难受了。

Nurse: OK, Mr. Gu, now I'm going to remove your pillow. If you are scared, just close your eyes, relax and take a deep breath, we will finish soon.

护士: 好的。顾先生,现在枕头先给您去掉了。如果害怕就闭上眼睛。放轻松点,深呼吸,很快就完成了。

Mr. Gu: Please be as gentle as you can.

顾先生: 请尽量轻点。

Doctor: We will. Nurse Wang, please pay attention to the patient's vital signs, if his blood oxygen **saturation** goes down to 90%, please let me know.

医生：我们会尽量轻柔的。王护士，请注意患者的生命体征变化，血氧饱和度低于 90% 报告一下。

Nurse: OK, we are ready now.

护士：好的。都准备好了。

Doctor: OK, give me the **sample container**. I will collect the deep lung sputum for testing.

医生：好的，先接痰标本管。留取深部痰培养。

Nurse: Here you are. The patient's saturation now is 95%.

护士：给您。患者目前血样饱和度 95%。

(5 minutes later)

（5 分钟后）

Nurse: The saturation has gone down to 90% and his heart rate is up to 130 beats/min.

护士：患者血氧降至 90%。心率升到 130 次 / 分。

Doctor: Let's take a rest. Please use the non-invasive ventilation as soon as I remove the bronchofibroscope.

医生：让患者休息一下。取出支纤镜后予盖回面罩无创通气。

Nurse: OK, I'm ready.

王护士：好的，已经准备好了。

(3 minutes later, the doctor starts again, and after another 10 minutes, the treatment is finished.)

（3 分钟后医生继续开始，10 分钟后治疗结束。）

Doctor: Mr. Gu, we're finished. How are you feeling now?

医生：顾先生，已经做完了。现在感觉怎么样？

Mr. Gu: I can breathe better now.

顾先生：呼吸通畅了许多。

Nurse: That's good. For 2 hours you can't eat anything. After two hours, you can drink some water or eat some cool porridge first before you return to a full diet.

护士：那就好，但这两个小时内先不要吃东西。2 个小时候后再喝点粥之类温凉的半流质或流质的食物。

Mr. Gu: OK, thank you very much.

顾先生：好的，谢谢你们。

Part Three　Words and Phrases

第三部分　单词和短语

antibiotics [ˌæntɪbaɪˈɑtɪks] *n.*［药］抗生素；抗生学

【例句】So I gave her antibiotics. 于是我给她开了抗生素。

bronchofibroscope *n.* 纤维支纤镜

hydrochloride [ˌhaɪdrəˈkloraɪd] *n.* 盐酸盐；盐酸化物；氢氯化物

【例句】Fenfluramine hydrochloride is an appetite inhibitor, a major role in the central nervous system. 盐酸芬氟拉明是一种食欲抑制剂，主要作用于中枢神经系统。

inhalation [ˌɪnhəˈleʃən] *n.* 吸入；吸入药剂

【例句】Infection results from inhalation of contaminated water sprays or mists. 吸入污染的水雾或气雾可造成感染。

sample [ˈsæmpl] *vt.* 取样；尝试；抽样检查 *n.* 样品；样本；例子；(Sample) 人名；(英) 桑普尔 *adj.* 试样的，样品的；作为例子的

【例句】Results of the sample must be translated. 取样检查的结果必须附加说明。

container [kənˈtenɚ] *n.* 集装箱；容器

【例句】He drained all the old oil out of the container. 他把容器里积存的油全部倒出来了。

saturation [ˈsætʃəˈreʃən] *n.* 饱和；色饱和度；浸透；磁化饱和

【例句】The saturation and lightness of light also affect our perceptions. 饱和度和亮度也影响到我们的感觉。

（胡亚南　王芳芳）

Chapter Twenty-One   TCM Treatment

第二十一章
中医治疗

Part One   Case Presentation

Mr. Zhang, 66-year-old, is retired cadre who is hospitalized with **hemiplegia** caused by stroke. A relative of the patient recounted what happened the day of the stroke. One day in the early summer, the weather was stuffy. The patient suddenly passed out and collapsed when he was watering flowers in the backyard. After being send to hospital immediately for emergency treatment, **intracerebral** hemorrhage (ICH) on the left side was discovered in his CT scan. Vital signs of the patient stabilized after six days of emergency treatment. Examination shows that the patient is conscious, but his language is not very clear. He also has facial paralysis and can not frown. The patient is paralyzed on the right side of his body with high-level hemiplegia. By diagnostic method of **inspection**, it is observed that the patient shows apparent pain, pale tongue and thin coating. Using the diagnostic method of **pulse-taking**, he is found to have a thin pulse string in both hands. Activating qi and collateral method as well as promoting circulation and removing stasis method are the major treatment methods. For TCM treatment acupuncture is mainly carried out in this case, and below is the conversation between the doctor and patient during the first acupuncture treatment.

第一部分 病 案 介 绍

张先生,退休干部,66 岁,因中风半身不遂收住医院。患者家属代诉:入夏的一日,天气闷热,患者在家中后院浇花时突然昏迷,即送医院进行抢救。经头颅 CT 检查显示:左侧颅内出血,经抢救治疗六日后,患者生命体征稳定。专科检查:患者神志清醒,语言欠清,口眼㖞斜,不能皱眉。右半身不遂,重度瘫痪。望诊:痛苦面容,舌淡苔薄。切脉:双手弦细。治疗以益气通络,活血化瘀为主。中医采用针灸治疗,以下是医生和患者在第一次针灸治疗时的对话。

Part Two   Dialogue

第二部分   对   话

Doctor: Good morning, Mr. Zhang. My name is Wang Bin, I will be looking after you, you can call me Xiao Wang. You will receive acupuncture treatment from today, how do you feel?

医生：早上好，张先生，我是您的主治医生王兵，您可以叫我小王。从今天起，我们就要开始针灸治疗了，感觉如何？

Mr. Zhang: Hello, Doctor Wang. I ... I am nervous. I'm feeling down ... can not move ... Hope acupuncture helps me ... Sorry to trouble you.

张先生：您好，王医生。我……紧张，心情低落，行动不便，希望针灸可以缓解我的病……麻烦您了。

Doctor: Don't be nervous. Take it easy. Compared with West medicine, TCM is more effective in treating **cardio-cerebro-vascular** diseases and nervous system diseases. What's more, there are no side effects.

医生：不要紧张，放松心态，与西医相比，中医在心脑血管疾病和神经系统疾病方面的疗效更为显著，且无任何副作用。

Doctor: So, no worries! We have successfully cured many patients like you in clinical therapy.

医生：请您放心！像您这样的患者，我们临床治疗的成功案例有很多。

Mr. Zhang: ... How long until I see the effects?

张先生：……多久会有疗效？

Doctor: Well, it depends on your physical condition and **rehabilitation** therapy. Generally, it will work after one course of treatment.

医生：这得根据您的身体状况和每天康复练习情况，一般一个疗程会见效。

Mr. Zhang: Then how long is it?

张先生：一个疗程是多久？

Doctor: One course is a treatment duration of ten days, then you will have a rest. Three days later, we'll continue the treatment with the next course. So, we'll get started now. Have you had breakfast?

医生：十天为一个疗程，休息三天，再继续下一疗程的治疗。那我们今天就开始吧。早饭吃过了吗？

Mr. Zhang: Yes. The nurse said, "Light diet, less oily dishes" ... I had porridge and steamed bread this morning.

张先生：吃过了，护士嘱咐：饮食清淡，少油腻……早上吃的稀饭和馒头。

Doctor: OK, you'd better not fast before receiving acupuncture. Relax, stay calm, and avoid burnout. Now, let's begin. Please lie on your back slowly. We will administer **clinostatism** acupuncture according to your condition.

医生：好的，针灸治疗前一定不要空腹。精神放松，情绪平稳，避免劳累。那我们开始吧，您缓慢仰卧，根据病情，我们采取卧位针刺。

Mr. Zhang: OK.

张先生：好。

Doctor: (Sterilized cotton is used before the acupuncture treatment) Firstly, I'll give you scalp acupuncture. Head acupoints on language and motor function regions are good for recovery of language and limb-function. What do you feel?

医生：（扎针前，医生在患者施针部位用酒精棉消毒）我们先在头部取穴，头部取语言区、运动区的穴位；有利于语言功能的恢复和肢体运动能力的恢复。有感觉吗？

Mr. Zhang: Pain ...

张先生：疼……

Doctor: Relax! The more you relax, the less pain you will feel.

医生：放松！越放松，针刺疼痛感越不明显。

Mr. Zhang: OK ...

张先生：嗯……

Doctor: Now, I'll give you facial acupuncture. Take it easy! **Acupoints** ST6 Jiache, ST7 Xiaguan, ST4 Dicang are very effective in treating your facial paralysis.

医生：接下来我们开始面部施针了，不要紧张！颊车，下关，地仓穴都对你现在口眼㖞斜的症状十分有效。

Doctor: Now, I'll give you acupuncture in your limbs. Try to hold on and keep still. LI10 Shousanli, ST36 Zusanli, SP6 Sanyinjiao, SP9 Yinlingquan and GB34 Yanglingquan are major acupoints for recovering movement in your limbs. How do you feel right now?

医生：现在我们开始四肢取穴位了，尽量保持不动。手三里，足三里，三阴交，阴陵泉，阳陵泉等都是主要穴位，对你肢体运动功能的康复很有帮助。现在感觉如何？

Mr. Zhang: Less pain, but sore and numb.

张先生：疼减轻了，但是感觉酸、胀。

Doctor: That's good, if you feel it. Acupuncture works! No worries, just let yourself get used to it slowly. We will stop here today. The nurse will come and remove the needles in half an hour. Be careful not to catch cold in case cold-dampness and pathogenic factors enter your body. See you tomorrow then.

医生：有针感说明穴位正确,是针灸的有效反应! 不要担心。慢慢适应。好的,今天施针就到这里,半小时后护士来取针。注意不要吹凉风,避免寒湿邪气入侵。今天就这样,明天我们继续。

Mr. Zhang: Thank you, Dr. Wang.

张先生：谢谢王医生。

Doctor: You are welcome. You can ring the bell if you need any help. See you.

医生：不客气,有问题可以按铃呼叫护士。明天见。

Part Three　Words and Phrases

第三部分　单词和词组

hemiplegia [ˌhɛmɪˈplidʒɪə] *n.* [内科]偏瘫,半身麻痹 [中医]半身不遂

【例句】Results: Cure 13 cases, low-level hemiplegia 3 cases, lose language ability 2 cases. 结果：所有收入病例治愈 13 例,轻度偏瘫 3 例,2 例失语。

intracerebral [ˌɪntrəsəˈribrəl] *adj.* 大脑内的

【例句】Infarction is the most common cause of secondary intracerebral hemorrhage. 脑梗死是继发性颅内出血最常见的诱因。

inspection [ɪnˈspɛkʃən] *n.* [中医]望诊

pulse-taking [ˈpʌlsˌtekɪŋ] *n.* [中医]脉诊

cardio-cerebro-vascular　心脑血管病

rehabilitation [ˌrihəˌbɪlɪˈteʃn] *n.* 康复,复原

【例句】They need extra attention during early rehabilitation. 他们需要在早期康复时期给予特别的关注。

clinostatism [klaɪˈnɒstətɪzəm] *n.* 卧位

【例句】Objective: to investigate the best clinostatism in senile patient after lumbar puncture. 目的是探讨提高老年患者腰穿术后舒适且又安全的合适卧位。

acupoint [ˈækjʊˈpɔɪnt] *n.* 穴道,[中医]穴位

【例句】Cupping is the method of applying a cup in which a partial vacuum is created over an acupoint for therapeutic purpose. 拔罐法是指使罐紧吸于穴位上进行治疗的方法。

Phrases and Expressions

activating qi and collateral　益气通络

promoting circulation and removing stasis　活血化瘀

four diagnostic methods (inspection, auscultation and olfaction, inquiry, pulse-taking and palpation)　望闻问切

（赵晓燕）

第二十二章
术后病人换药（医生）

Background

A bone fracture is a medical condition in which there is a damage in the continuity of the bone. A bone fracture can be the result of high force impact or stress, or a minimal trauma injury as a result of certain medical conditions that weaken the bones, such as osteoporosis, bone cancer, or **osteogenesisimperfecta**, where the fracture is then properly termed a pathologic fracture. Although broken bone and bone break are common colloquialisms for a bone fracture, break is not a formal orthopedic term. A bone fracture may be diagnosed based on the history given and the physical examination performed. Radio graphic imaging is often performed, to confirm the diagnosis. Under certain circumstances, radiographic examination of the nearby joints is indicated in order to exclude dislocations and fracture-dislocations. In situations where projectional radiography alone is insufficient, computed tomography (CT) or magnetic resonance imaging (MRI) may be indicated.

骨折是指骨的连续性遭到破坏。骨折可能是由于某些疾病导致骨骼脆弱,如骨质疏松、骨癌、或成骨不全症,这些被称为病理性骨折。骨断或骨碎是骨折的口语表达,这些并不是正式的骨科术语。骨折的诊断基于特定的病史和检查。射线成像通常有助于确诊。在某些情况下,对骨折附近的关节进行射线检查,以排除脱位或明确断裂位置。在单纯 X 射线显示不清时,需要计算机断层摄影（CT）或核磁共振成像（MRI）。

Part One   Case Presentation

Mr.Zhang, 46 years old, was admitted to the hospital for "an hour of left leg pain caused by car accident". His lower limb X-ray showed his left fibula and tibia comminuted fracture. His surgeon gave him an initial fixation, and now he is in the preparation for a surgery.

At orthopedic unit, nurse Chen is taking care of patient Mr.Zhang who has **skeletal** traction on his left leg. Intern nurse Li follows nurse Chen delivering patient care.

第一部分 病案介绍

46岁的张先生因"车祸导致左腿疼痛1小时"入院。下肢X片显示左腓骨、胫骨粉碎性骨折。外科医生给予固定术后准备择期手术。

在医院整形外科病房，护士小陈照顾病人张先生。张先生的左腿上有骨牵引。实习护士小李跟随护士小陈为患者做护理。

Part Two　Dialogue

第二部分　对　话

Nurse Chen: Li, I'm going to do **pin care** of patient Mr. Zhang. You want to come with me?

陈护士：小李，我要去护理病人张先生。你要跟我来吗？

Nurse Li: Yes, thank you for asking me.

李护士：是的，谢谢你叫我。

Nurse Chen: You're welcome. I think it's good for you to learn about the traction and pin care. The patient had a car accident and had fraction of his **left tibia** and **fibula**. He is in skeletal traction. Come on, let's get the supplies.

陈护士：不客气。这是个好机会让你了解牵引护理。这个病人发生了车祸，左胫骨和腓骨骨折，目前在行骨牵引术。我们来准备一些物品吧。

Nurse Li: What supplies do we need for the pin care?

李护士：我们需要准备什么物品？

Nurse Chen: I usually take a wrap like Kerlix or conform, some 2 by 2 sterile gauze sponges, betadine swabs, sterile saline, and bandages. I always have tape and scissors in my pocket. Get everything? OK, let's go to the patient room.

(Nurse Chen and Li walk into patient Zhang's room.)

陈护士：我通常需要2×2无菌纱布海绵、棉签、无菌生理盐水，绷带。我总是有胶带和剪刀在口袋里。都准备齐了？好的，我们去病人的房间。

（陈护士和李护士走进病人张先生的房间。）

Nurse Chen: Hi, Mr. Zhang, how are you doing?

陈护士：您好，张先生，感觉怎么样？

Mr. Zhang: I'm OK. How are you?

张先生：我很好，你好吗？

Nurse Chen: Pretty good. We are going to change the dressing at pin sites. Li is a nursing student. She is going to help with the dressing change. Is that OK with you?

陈护士：很好。我们要在牵引处换药。小李是一个护理实习生。她将帮助换药。这样可以吗？

Mr. Zhang: No problem.

张先生：没问题。

Nurse Chen: Thank you, Mr. Zhang. Li, let's take off the old dressings. Put on your gloves, Li. Mr. Zhang, I'm taking off the dressings. Are you having any pain at the pin sites?

陈护士：谢谢您，张先生。小李，我们撤走旧的敷料。戴上你的手套。张先生，我将揭开敷料，疼吗？

Mr. Zhang: A little bit.

张先生：有点儿疼。

Nurse Chen: OK. The dressings are off. Now, we need to inspect the sites for signs of infection. What are the signs and symptoms of infection?

陈护士：好的。现在我们需要检查感染的迹象。感染的症状和体征是什么？

Nurse Li: Signs are redness, swelling drainage, and fever. Symptoms are pain and chills.

李护士：发红、肿胀和发烧。症状是疼痛和寒战。

Nurse Chen: Very good. And Mr. Zhang, do you feel any discomfort at your pin sites?

陈护士：很好。张先生您在牵引部位感到任何不适吗？

Mr. Zhang: Some discomfort. Other than that, I'm OK.

张先生：有些不适。不过我很好。

Nurse Chen: The sites look good, too. You have been well taken care of. All right. Now we are going to clean the sites. We need to do the cleaning really well.

陈护士：伤口看起来不错。您的伤口护理得很好。好吧。现在我们将要清洁伤口。我们需要做彻底清洁。

Nurse Li: What do we use?

小李：我们使用什么？

Nurse Chen: Betadine swabs. You watch me clean this pin, and I'll let you do the next one.

陈护士：碘伏棉签。你先看我示范，然后你做下一个。

(Chen cleans a pin site with a betadine swab. She starts by swabbing around the pin and then goes outward with a circular motion.)

（陈护士用碘伏棉签以打钉处为中心，以打圈的方式由内向外消毒，李护士按陈护士示范的方式做了一遍。）

Nurse Chen: Good. Make sure you never ever use the same applicator used on one site for another pin site care. That will cause cross contamination. In fact, you should not go over any area twice with the same swab. If debri remains after cleaning with the first swab, discard it and use a fresh swab to complete the cleaning.

陈护士：很好。确保你不要使用相同的棉签清洗同一个伤口。这将引起交叉污染。清洁后丢弃棉签，用干净的棉签完成清洗。事实上，你不应该用同一个棉签接触任何一个区域两次。如果使用一根棉签清洗后，伤口的碎屑仍在，扔掉这根棉签，再使用另一根新的完成清洁。

(Chen and Li clean all the pin sites.)

（陈护士和李护士清洁所有伤口。）

Nurse Chen: There might be some areas on the leg that are not clean; we can use sterile saline to clean them. Just try to provide as clean an environment as possible to reduce the chances of infection.

陈护士：可能伤口的一些区域未清洗干净；我们可以用无菌生理盐水来清洗。尽可能提供干净的环境以减少感染的几率。

Nurse Li: Right.

李护士：对的。

Nurse Chen: Now we can put the dressing on. Be careful to put the cut edge right around the pin, and then we add the bandage on top. Looks good, right?

陈护士：现在我们可以敷药。小心地把纱布放在伤口处，然后加上绷带。看起来不错，对吧？

Nurse Li: Yes.

李护士：是的。

Nurse Chen: Now I tape it nicely.

陈护士：现在我绑好绷带。

Nurse Li: We don't put **antibiotic ointment** on the pin site?

李护士：我们不涂抗生素软膏吗？

Nurse Chen: At our hospital, we do not recommend putting ointment on if the pin site doesn't show signs of infection. If an antibiotic ointment is necessary, we will ask the doctor to prescribe it. But you might see other hospital use ointment.

陈护士：在我们医院，如果伤口没有感染的迹象，不使用抗生素。如果有必要，我们会要求医生开抗生素软膏。但是你可能会看到其他医院会使用抗生素软膏。

Nurse Li: Got it.

李护士：明白了。

Nurse Chen: Do you think you can dress the other one? I will watch you do it. Go ahead.

陈护士：你认为你能给另一边换药吗？来吧，我看着你做。

(The traction pin care continues.)

（继续牵引伤口的护理。）

Part Three   Words and Phrases

第三部分　单词和短语

osteogenesisimperfectan　*n.* 成骨不全症

skeletal ['skɛlətl] *adj.* 骨骼的，像骨骼的；骸骨的；骨瘦如柴的

【例句】So, how do we figure out first how to draw the skeletal structure of this molecule here?

那么，我们如何来解决它，首先是如何画出这个分子的骨架结构？

tibia　*n.* 胫骨

fibula　*n.* 腓骨

antibiotic ointment　*n.* 抗生素软膏

pin care　*n.* 钢针（牵引用）护理

Phrases and Expressions

be based on ...　根据；以……为基础

in order to ...　为了……

put on　戴上

（毛　帅　何建卓）

第二十三章
医生查房

Part One   Case Presentation

Mr. Li was admitted to the hospital for the 2-hour acutely right lower quadrant pain. He has hypertension history. After the medical check up, doctor found that he had abdominal muscle tension and board like rigidity. The CT test result showed that he might has appendicitis with perforation. Immediately started laparotomy and turned him to ICU after the surgery. The attending doctor inspected him in the next day.

第一部分   病 案 介 绍

李先生因"突发右下腹疼痛2小时"入院。既往高血压病史。医生检查时发现腹肌紧张、板状腹,行CT检查提示阑尾炎并穿孔。立即行剖腹探查术,术后转入重症医学科。第二天主管医生查房。

Part Two   Dialogue

第二部分   对　　话

Dialogue 1

Nurse: You look much better today.

护士：您今天看起来好一些了。

Mr.Li: Yes, but lying in bed all day, I feel uncomfortable all over.

李先生：是的,不过整天躺着我觉得全身不舒服。

Nurse: First, sit on the edge of the bed and if you don't feel dizzy then you can get out of bed today.

护士：您今天可以下床了，但在下床前先要在床边坐坐，没有头晕才能下床。

Mr.Li: But I feel distended in the abdomen.

李先生：不过我感到腹胀。

Nurse: Did you pass any wind by rectum?

护士：有排气吗？

Mr.Li: No.

李先生：没有。

Nurse: You can lie on your side more often, and if the wound does not hurt, you can get out of bed and walk around, that will help peristalsis of the intestine which will help to pass gas and lessen distension.

护士：可以多翻身，如果伤口不疼可下床活动，那样有助于恢复肠蠕动，使气体排出减轻腹胀。

Mr. Li: The wound is painful and the **sputum** is difficult to **expectorate**.

李先生：伤口疼，而且有痰又难咳出来。

Nurse: You should sit up. That will help your deep breathing, and help you to expectorate and prevent the sputum from accumulating in your lungs to cause **pneumonia**.

护士：您应该坐起来，那样可以帮助您深呼吸，使痰容易咳出，以防痰积在肺内引起肺炎。

Mr. Li: All right.

李先生：好的。

Nurse: Did you drink any water?

护士：您喝过水了吗？

Mr. Li: Yes.

李先生：喝过了。

Nurse: Do you feel distended and nausea?

护士：您感觉胃胀和恶心吗？

Mr. Li: No.

李先生：没有。

Nurse: That's good. You can start on a fluid diet and congee in two days.

护士：那很好，您可以开始吃流质，过两天吃稀饭。

Mr. Li: Thank you.

李先生：谢谢。

Mr. Li: How long must I stay in hospital?

李先生: 我住院还需多久?

Nurse: You can go home in about a week.

护士: 一个星期左右便可出院了。

Nurse: Good morning, doctor.

护士: 医生,早上好。

Doctor: Good morning. How is the patient after surgery?

医生: 早晨好,病人手术后情况如何?

Nurse: The patient has a slight pain in the wound. Some blood has been oozing from the draining wound, the dressing has been changed once.

护士: 伤口有点疼。伤口引流有些渗血,换过一次敷料。

Doctor: That's good.

医生: 那很好。

Nurse: Does he still need intravenous infusion and **penicillin**?

护士: 静脉输液和青霉素是否继续给?

Doctor: Yes.

医生: 继续。

Dialogue2

Nurse: Good morning, Mr.Li. It's time for me to give you intravenous infusion.

护士: 李先生,上午好! 该给您输液了。

Mr. Li: Excuse me, could you tell me about the use of the IV fluids?

李先生: 对不起,您能告诉我输这些液体的作用吗?

Nurse: Of course. The fluids can provide energy for you and prevent you from electrolytic imbalances after operation.

护士: 当然可以。输入的液体能为您提供能量,还可预防术后电解质失衡。

Mr. Li: Would you please let the fluid drop more quickly?

李先生: 请您把液体滴速调快点儿好吗?

Nurse: Your IV fluids must be given slowly so as not to overload you.

护士: 那不可以的。您的静脉输液必须慢速,不然会增加心脏负荷。

Part Three　Words and Phrases

第三部分　单词和短语

sputum ['spjʊtəm] *n.*［生理］痰；唾液

【例句】TB is usually diagnosed by looking at a sputum smear under a microscope. 通常，结核病是采用痰液涂片镜检的方式诊断的。

expectorate [ɪk'spɛktəret] *vt.* 咳出痰；吐唾液；咯血 *vi.* 咳出痰等；吐唾液；咯血

【例句】Do not expectorate on the sidewalks. 不要在人行道上吐痰。

penicillin [ˌpɛnɪ'sɪlɪn] *n.* 青霉素

【例句】Most bacterial infections can be treated with antibiotics such as penicillin, discovered decades ago. 大多数细菌感染可以用抗生素治疗，如早在几十年前发现的青霉素。

Phrases and Expressions

feel distended in the abdomen　腹胀

lie on your side　翻身

（毛　帅）

第二十四章

解释检验结果

Part One   Case Presentation

Mrs. Wang, 84-years-old, is hospitalized with "recurrent dizziness that is last for 20 years and has been aggravated over a week". She was diagnosed with hypertension when she was admitted for dizziness 20 years ago. The blood pressure (BP) was high up to 190/100 mmHg once, which is under control by taking Extended Release Nifedipine Tablets combined with hydrochlorothiazide. Occasionally, mood swings or weather changes can lead to dizziness attack, which will be relieved by medicine. She complained that dizziness reappeared after a quarrel with neighbors one week ago, accompanied by chest tightness and dazzle, and the self BP measurement was 210/120 mmHg. She denied nausea and vomiting, palpitations, shortness of breath, abdominal pain and edema of lower limbs. She was transmitted to CCU from outpatient department with the diagnosis of "hypertension emergency". The symptoms were relieved by controlling the blood with sodium nitroprusside in CCU, and the fundus examination, cardiac color Doppler ultrasound, renal color Doppler ultrasound and routine biochemical examination were given by the CCU doctor. The competent doctor is explaining the results of the related examination to Mrs. Wang during the rounds.

第一部分   病案介绍

王女士,84 岁,因"反复头晕 20 年加重 1 周余"入院。20 年前因头晕住院治疗,发现血压高,最高达 190/100mmHg,长期服用硝苯地平缓释片联合氢氯噻嗪控制血压。情绪波动或天气变化时偶有头晕发作,服药后可以缓解。1 周前与邻居吵架后头晕再发,自测血压 210/120mmHg,伴胸闷不适,目眩,无恶心呕吐,无心悸气促,无腹胀腹痛,无双下肢浮肿。门诊以"高血压急症"收入 CCU。CCU 医生予硝普钠控制血压后症状缓解,行眼底镜检查、心脏彩超、肾脏彩超以及常规生化等检查。查房时主管医生和王奶奶讲述相关检查结果。

Part Two   Dialogue

第二部分   对   话

(The patient looks at the lab results)

（病人在看她的实验室检查结果）

Mrs. Wang: My **LDL cholesterol** is 190, and the normal is less than 100.

王女士：我的低密度脂蛋白胆固醇是 190，正常的不到 100。

Doctor: You notice that, ha?

医生：嗯，您也注意到了。

Mrs. Wang: What does it mean? Is it serious?

王女士：它意味着什么？这很严重吗？

Doctor: It can become serious. If your LDL is high, cholesterol will **accumulate** in your blood vessels and build up fatty **plaques**.

医生：会变得严重。如果你的低密度脂蛋白胆固醇高，就会存积在你的血管里并形成脂肪斑块。

Mrs. Wang: How serious could it be?

王女士：它会进展严重到什么程度？

Doctor: Over the years, it can make your blood vessels narrower and less flexible. If your blood vessel is very narrow, the blood flow through it is limited. This can cause angina. If the blood vessel is completely blocked by the plaque, or a blood clot forms on the plaque, a heart attack, stroke, or other serious condition may result.

医生：再经过几年，它可以使您的血管变得狭窄并且不再那么柔软。如果您的血管非常狭窄，血流就会受到限制。这可能会导致心绞痛。如果血管完全被脂肪斑块或血块堵塞，会导致心脏病、中风或者其他更严重的后果。

Mrs. Wang: That's bad.

王女士：哦，那太糟糕了。

Doctor: Right. That's why LDL is also called the bad cholesterol.

医生：是的，这就是为什么低密度脂蛋白也被称为坏胆固醇。

Mrs. Wang: What treatment would I need, then?

王女士：那么我需要什么治疗呢？

Doctor: To begin with, you will need to make life style changes regarding diet and exercise. Next, you will need medications. I have already prescribed **lipitor** for you. You are going to start to take it today.

医生：首先，您需要改变饮食和运动方式。接下来，您需要药物治疗。我为您开了立普妥。您今天要开始服用它。

Mrs. Wang: Is it a pill?

王女士：那是药片吗？

Doctor: Yes, it's a medication that's clinically proven to lower cholesterol levels.

医生：是的，它是一种药物，临床上被证明能降低胆固醇。

Mrs. Wang: OK.

王女士：好的。

Doctor: And, as I told you in addition to taking medications, you will have to make some dietary changes and even life style changes that will be good for your heart health and overall well-being.

医生：除了我告诉你的服药外，你必须做出一些饮食方面的改变，甚至是生活方式变化，将有利于心脏和整体健康。

Mrs. Wang: What do I need to do?

王女士：我需要做些什么？

Doctor: Limit fatty food, fast food, and fried food; limit processed food and high sugar food; use **olive** oil for cooking ...

医生：限制高脂肪食品、快餐、油炸，腌制食品和高糖食物摄入，使用橄榄油做饭……等等。

Mrs. Wang: OK, but no matter what, I have to eat less fat, right?

王女士：好吧，但是无论怎么，我还是需要少量脂肪的对吗？

Doctor: You are so right.

医生：嗯，确实是这样。

Part Three　Words and Phrases

第三部分　单词和短语

cholesterol [kəˈlɛstərɒl] *n.* 胆固醇

【例句】If it does, you should discuss with your physician about other approaches to cholesterol control. 若确实如此，您应该与您的医生讨论其他控制胆固醇方法。

plaque [plæk] *n.* 斑块

【例句】These minerals form crystals and harden the plaque structure. 这些矿物质形成了菌斑的结晶变硬的结构。

lipitor   *n.* 立普妥（药品名，降血脂药）

olive ['ɑlɪv] *n.* 橄榄，橄榄树

【例句】I even fry sage to crispness in olive oil and shake on some sea salt as a reminder of summers in Italy. 我甚至把鼠尾草用橄榄油炸得松脆，然后再上面撒一些海盐，作为对在意大利度过的夏天的一种怀念。

LDL=low density lipoprotein   *n.* 低密度脂蛋白

accumulate [əˈkjumjələt] *vi.* 积聚；堆积

【例句】Not only did I accumulate important experience for job, but also realize what I want to be in the future. 不仅是因为我积累了工作经验，而且我意识到了我未来将从事的工作。

Phrases and Expressions

in addition to   除……之外
no matter what   无论怎么

（毛　帅　谭益冰）

Chapter Twenty-Five   Child Care

第二十五章
儿童保健

Background

Child care or childcare, child minding, or preschool is the caring for and supervision of a child or children, usually from age six weeks to age one. Child care is the action or skill of looking after children by a day-care center, babysitter, or other providers. Child care is a broad topic covering a wide **spectrum** of **contexts**, activities, social and cultural **conventions**, and **institutions**. **The majority of** child care institutions that are available require that child care providers have **extensive** training in **first aid** and are **CPR certified**. In addition, background checks, drug testing at all centers, and **reference verification** are normally a requirement. Child care can cost up to $15,000 for one year in the United States. The average annual cost of full-time care for an infant in center-based care ranges from $4,863 in Mississippi to $16,430 in Massachusetts. Early child care is a very important and often overlooked **component** of child development. Child care providers are our children's first teachers, and therefore **play an integral role** in our systems of early childhood education. Quality care from a young age can **have a huge impact on** the future successes of children.

儿童保育、儿童保健或学前教育通常是指照顾六周到一岁的儿童。儿童保健是托儿所、保姆或其他人照看孩子的行为或技能。儿童保健是一个宽泛的主题,涉及广泛的背景、活动、社会和文化习俗。大多数儿童保健机构可以要求孩子保健提供者有广泛的急救和心肺复苏培训认证。此外背景调查、药物测试和参考验证通常是必需的。在美国儿童保健成本高达 15 000 美元 / 年。全职照顾一个婴儿的年平均费用,在密西西比州约 4863 美元,而马萨诸塞州约 16 430 美元。儿童早期保健是一项非常重要但是常被忽视的内容。儿童保健提供者是我们孩子的第一任老师,因此在我们的幼儿教育体系中扮演着不可或缺的角色。护理质量可以对孩子未来的成功产生巨大影响。

Part One   Case Presentation

Ms. Zhang is a young mother. According to the doctor's request, Ms. Zhang takes her child to the pediatric clinic for health care. Here is a conversation between Ms. Zhang and the pediatrician.

第一部分　病 案 介 绍

张女士是一个年轻的妈妈,按照医生要求,张女士带着孩子到儿科门诊做保健。以下是张女士和儿科保健医生的对话。

Part Two   Dialogue

第二部分　对　　话

Doctor: The baby has a heart murmur, but this may be normal. Does he seem to be pretty active?

医生:这个婴儿心脏有杂音,但杂音可能是正常的。他看起来很活泼?

Ms. Zhang: Oh, yes.

张女士:哦,是的。

Doctor: Does he ever turn blue after eating or after crying?

医生:他吃奶或哭闹后有发青紫的现象吗?

Ms. Zhang: Well, I haven't noticed anything like that.

张女士:哦,我没有注意到那样的情况。

Doctor: Does he seem to get tired very often?

医生:他经常显得疲劳吗?

Ms. Zhang: When he cries a lot he does.

张女士:当他哭多了就显得疲劳。

Doctor: We'll watch this condition. Is he on any other food than the formula?

医生:我们要注意这种情况。他除了吃配方奶以外还吃其他食物吗?

Ms. Zhang: No.

张女士:不吃。

Doctor: How much formula is he taking?

医生:他吃多少配方奶?

Ms. Zhang: Five ounces.

张女士：5 盎司（142 克）。

Doctor: I mean the total, in a day. Is he up to a quart?

医生：我的意思是一天的总量是多少？能吃 1 夸脱（1.14 升）吗？

Ms. Zhang: Just about that.

张女士：差不多 1 夸脱。

Doctor: Well, we usually don't like them to get more than a quart a day. We'll start him on some solids. He's gaining weight nicely, I see...No other problems?

医生：呃，我们一般不愿意让他们一天吃 1 夸脱以上。要开始给他吃些固体食物。他的体重增长得很好，……没有其他问题了吧？

Ms. Zhang: I don't think so.

张女士：没有了。

Part Three　Words and Phrases

第三部分　单词和短语

spectrum ['spɛktrəm] *n.* 光谱；频谱；范围；余象

context ['kantɛkst] *n.* 环境；上下文；来龙去脉

a wide spectrum of contexts　广泛的背景

convention [kən'vɛnʃən] *n.* 大会；[法]惯例；约定；协定；习俗

【例句】Originality often triumphs over convention. 创意常常战胜惯例。

institution [ˌɪnstɪ'tuʃən] *n.* 制度；建立；公共机构；习俗

【例句】I think that everyone should get married at least once, so you can see what a silly, outdated institution it is. 我认为每个人都应该至少结一次婚，这样你就能看到它是一个多么愚蠢、过时的制度。

extensive [ɪk'stɛnsɪv] *adj.* 广泛的；大量的；广阔的

【例句】His extensive experience in other parts of Asia helped him to overcome cultural barriers. 他在亚洲其他地区的丰富经验帮助他克服了文化障碍。

CPR　*abbr.* 心肺复苏术（cardiopulmonary resuscitation）

【例句】The experts said performing CPR in inappropriate cases could result in a distressing and undignified death. 专家说，在不适当的情况下实施 CPR 可能会导致痛苦和不尊严的死亡。

certified ['sɝtəˌfaɪd] *adj.* 被证明的；有保证的；具有证明文件的

CPR certified　持有心肺复苏证明

reference ['rɛfrəns] *n.* 参考,参照;涉及,参考书目;介绍信;证明书

【例句】The above views may or may not be correct, they are only for your reference. 以上观点可能是正确的,也可能不是正确的,只是供你参考。

verification [ˌvɛrɪfɪ'keʃən] *n.* 确认,查证;核实

【例句】Then there's the question of who would provide the verification data for the forecasts. 然后是谁将为预测提供验证数据的问题。

component [kəm'ponənt] *adj.* 组成的,构成的 *n.* 成分;组件;元件

【例句】But what if none of them contain the component that you need? 但是,如果它们之中没有一个包含你需要的成分怎么办?

formula ['fɔrmjələ] *n.* [数]公式,准则;配方;婴儿食品

【例句】Australia and the UK have set limits on the sale of baby formula. 澳大利亚和英国已经限制了婴儿配方奶粉的销售。

Phrases and Expressions

play an integral role   扮演着不可或缺的角色

turn blue   发青紫

heart murmur   心脏杂音

first aid   急救、急救护理

the majority of   ……的大多数(反义词 minority)

have a huge impact on   对……有巨大影响

（毛　帅）

Chapter Twenty-Six   Health Education (Nurse)

第二十六章
出院病人的健康宣教（护士）

Part One   Case Presentation

Mr. Zhang, 65-year-old, has been admitted because of "repeated stuffy chest pain lasting for half a year, which has become serious in the past 2 hours". His heart rate is 40 beats/min, blood pressure is 100/50 mmHg, **ECG indicates** acute myocardial infarction. Mr. Zhang has been transferred to the **Percutaneous** Department for **coronary angiography**, and had one **stent inserted** in his right coronary **artery**. Mr. Zhang felt the pain disperse after the surgery, and 3 days later, the patient is about to be discharged from the hospital, the nurse in charge of his case is giving him some basic health education.

第一部分   病 案 介 绍

张先生,65岁,因"反复胸前区闷痛半年,加重2小时"入院,心率40次/分,血压100/50mmHg,心电图提示急性心肌梗死,紧急送介入室行冠脉造影术并在右冠状动脉置入支架一个,术后患者胸闷痛缓解,术后第3天患者准备出院,主管护士为其做出院宣教。

Part Two   Dialogue

第二部分   对   话

Nurse: Mr. Zhang, your doctor is about to discharge you today.
护士:张先生,您好。医生让您今天出院。

Mr. Zhang: Yes, Dr. Li told me this morning when we did bed rounds.

张先生：是的,李医生早上查房的时候和我说了。

Nurse: Congratulations, Mr. Zhang. There are some things you need to know before your discharge.

护士：恭喜您。您要出院了,和您再交代一下注意事项。

Mr. Zhang: OK, what are they ?

张先生：好的, 是什么呢?

Nurse: You know you had AMI, and you have had one stent inserted. When you are at home, you need to take your medication regularly as **per** the doctor's order. Do you know what medications you need to take, and what you need to pay attention to?

护士：您已经知道自己有急性心肌梗死,目前放了支架,出院之后,第一就是要按照医生的要求服药。您知道自己这几天都吃什么药吗? 要注意什么吗?

Mr. Zhang: Yes, I know, there are aspirin and **plavix**. I need to pay attention to any **hemorrhagic** symptoms, also the color of my stool.

张先生：嗯,知道,有阿司匹林,波立维。要注意一些出血的症状,还有观察自己大便的颜色.

Nurse: Yes, very good. Also you should never stop the medication yourself, and if you have any inquiries about your medication please contact your doctor.

护士：嗯,非常好。出院后不要随便自己停药,有疑问时及时就医。

Mr. Zhang: Okay, I will.

张先生：好的,知道了。

Nurse: If you have **chest** pain after discharge, try to take nitroglycerin **sublingually**. If it doesn't work after 3~5 minutes, you can take another one. If it still doesn't work, you need to go to hospital as soon as you can.

护士：出院后如果有胸闷痛,可以舌下含服随身携带的硝酸甘油,如果 3~5 分钟不能缓解可以再服一粒,持续不能缓解记得赶紧去医院。

Mr. Zhang: OK, I see. I will carry nitroglycerin with me all the time.

张先生：嗯,出门我都会随身带着药。

Nurse: You also need to follow a good diet. Eat low calorie food, high cellulose vegetables, which will help you have regular bowel movements.

护士：出院之后要注意饮食调节。进食一些低脂、低胆固醇、低盐、高纤维素的食物,保持大便通畅。

Mr. Zhang: Yes, I will pay attention to that.

张先生：嗯,我会注意的。

Nurse: You need to develop some good habit. For example, give up smoking, go to sleep earlier, try to stay in a good mood.

护士:注意调整自己一些习惯。比如戒烟、早睡,保持好心情。

Mr. Zhang: You are right. I will definitely quit smoking this time.

张先生:嗯,这次一定要把烟戒了。

Nurse: Here is our contact information. If you need any help, do not hesitate to contact us, and we will call you sometimes, too.

护士:这里有我们的联系方式,如果您需要帮助,请一定联系我们。我们也会定期电话随访您的情况。

Mr. Zhang: Thank you very much. This is a great help.

张先生:非常感谢,这个太有用了。

Part Three   Words and Phrases

第三部分   单词和短语

ECG [ˌiːsiːˈdʒiː] *abbr.* 心电图(Electrocardiograph)

【例句】Holter monitor. This portable ECG device can be worn for a day or more to record your heart's activity as you go about your routine. 动态心电图,这是一种可随身携带的心电图,可以在你正常生活时连续记录下几天内心脏的活动。

indicate ['ɪndɪket] *vt.* 表明;指出;预示;象征

【例句】Her face indicates her feelings. 她的表情表明了她的感觉。

sublingually   *adj.* 舌下的;舌下腺的

【例句】To observe the effects of methyl carprost suppository given sublingually on postpartum bleeding in normal parturients. 探讨舌下含服卡前列甲酯栓预防产后出血的效果。

stuffy ['stʌfi] *adj.* 闷热的;古板的;不通气的

【例句】The room was so stuffy that one could hardly breathe. 屋里太闷,憋得人透不过气来。

chest [tʃɛst] *n.* 胸,胸部;衣柜;箱子;金库

【例句】She snuggled up to his chest. 她偎依在他的胸前。

percutaneons   *adj.* 经皮的;经由皮肤的

coronary ['kɔrənɛri] *adj.* 冠的;冠状的;花冠的;冠状动脉或静脉的

【例句】In older people, the causes are the same as for other coronary problems: hypertension, high cholesterol and smoking. 在老年人身上,其病因和其他冠心病问题是相同的:高血压,高胆固醇和吸烟。

angiography [ænʤɪˈagrəfi] *n.* [特医]血管造影术;血管照相术;血管学;[特医]血管

造影法

【例句】One big advance has been in the use of computed tomography angiography. 其中一项已投入使用的进 展是计算机断层扫描血管造影术。

artery ['ɑrtəri] *n.* 动脉; 干道; 主流

【例句】Heart disease and artery disease will raise your risk of heart disease. 心脏病和动脉疾病会增加你患中风的风险。

stent [stent] *n.* ［医］斯滕特氏印模膏; 支架; 展伸;(Stent) 人名;(英) 斯滕特 *adj.* 扩张的

【例句】The tube is supported by a metallic support, or stent. 管腔内由金属支撑物或者支架支撑。

inserted [ɪn'səːtɪd] *adj.* 插入的;［生物］嵌入的; 著生的; 附着的

【例句】He inserted a letter into the misspelled word. 他在拼错的单词中插进了一个字母。

per [pɚ] *prep.* 每; 经; 按照; 每一 *n.*(Per) 人名;(德、挪、丹、瑞典) 佩尔

【例句】They are ramming their motorcycles on the expressway at 80 miles per hour. 他们正以每小时 80 英里的速度骑着摩托车在高速公路上疾驶。

plavix　*n.* 氯吡格雷(波立维)

hemorrhagic ['hemərædʒɪk] *adj.* 出血的

【例句】Cases are generally non-lethal but dengue occasionally results in a deadly hemorrhagic fever. 一般不会致死但是偶尔会引起致命的出血热。

cellulose ['sɛljulos] *n.* 纤维素;(植物的) 细胞膜质

【例句】Besides cellulose, there are hemicellulose and lignin. 除了纤维素, 还有半纤维素和木质素。

（胡亚南　王芳芳）

Chapter Twenty-Seven　Early Cardiac Rehabilitation Training Following PCI

第二十七章
经皮冠状动脉介入术后早期康复训练

Part One　Case Presentation

Mr. Zeng, a 48-year-old male, had been hospitalized with "chest distress with pain emanating to back and shoulder for 2 hours". The examinations showed that he might be suffering from an acute myocardial infarction, so he had emergency surgery immediately with an insertion of an **endovascular stent (percutaneous coronary intervention, PCI)** in the **left anterior descending coronary artery**. Admitted into the intensive care unit for better monitoring after the surgery, he was fully awake but tired and his vital signs were stable. The second day after surgery, early cardiac rehabilitation would be provided to Mr. Zeng after a full assessment of his safety.

第一部分　病案介绍

曾先生,48 岁,因为"胸闷痛伴有肩背部放射痛 2 小时"入院,检查考虑急性心肌梗死,立即行了急诊手术治疗,在左前降支放置支架一枚。术后转入重症医学科监护治疗,患者清醒,精神疲倦,生命体征暂时平稳。术后第 2 天,经评估安全,给予行早期心脏康复。

Part Two　Dialogue

第二部分　对　话

Nurse: Hello, Mr. Zeng. How do you do? Do you have any chest pain or any other discomfort?

护士: 曾先生,您好。现在有没胸闷痛等症状?

Mr. Zeng: No, I feel much better now. Thanks for asking.

曾先生: 已经没有了,感觉好很多。谢谢。

Nurse: Mr. Zeng, I suggest you to take up cardiac rehabilitation as soon as possible. I can teach you a traditional Chinese medicine training method called "Baduanjin continued regimen exercises".

护士: 曾先生,我建议您今早进行心脏康复训练。我可以教您八段锦序贯操,是一种中医康复方法。

Mr. Zeng: Is it suitable for me to do that considering I was told to rest in bed?

曾先生: 你们让我在床上休息,我现在适合做吗?

Nurse: Of course, Mr. Zeng. Now I am going to make a detailed introduction of this method. I suggest you to keep on practicing everyday even after you have been discharged, and we will keep following up your health condition and give you further instruction.

护士: 可以,我先给您详细介绍这种康复方法,建议您每天要坚持练,回家后也要坚持,我们会持续对您的健康状况进行跟进,并会对您进一步指导。

Mr. Zeng: Yes, please.

曾先生: 好的。

Nurse: As a traditional Chinese medicine health care practice method, Baduanjin is an important part of traditional Chinese medicine regimen and therapy. People can benefit physically and psychologically by practicing Baduanjin. It helps the circulation of qi and blood to improve the function of organs as well as emotional stability. According to the latest scientific research, Baduanjin meets the characteristics of **low-intensity** and long term **aerobic** exercise. It is really suitable following PCI.

护士: 八段锦是中医传统的保健术,是中医养生和治疗学的重要部分。八段锦不仅能够调心、调息、调形,改善气血运行,调节脏腑功能,疏导患者的不良情绪,而且符合现代研究低强度、长时间有氧运动的特点,非常适合您这种心肌梗死后的运动康复训练。

Mr. Zeng: It sounds great. I will stick to this.

曾先生: 听起来真不错,我会坚持练的。

Nurse: Since you should rest in bed, I suggest you practice the sitting version of Baduanjin. The standing version would apply to you after your condition becomes more stable.

护士: 您现在不能下床,先练习坐式八段锦。等您可以下床了,就练习立式八段锦。

Mr. Zeng: OK, so there are two versions, sitting and standing.

曾先生: 好的,还可以分坐式跟立式。

Nurse: Now I am going to show you a video of the sitting version. After you master it, you can do it all by yourself.

护士: 我现在先把这个疗法做给您看,然后就给您放视频,等您学会后,就不用看视频做了。

Mr. Zeng: What if I feel tired during the practice?

曾先生: 如果练习时感觉累呢?

Nurse: Mr. Zeng, don't worry about it. We will be monitoring your situation while you practice. If you feel uncomfortable, you can stop and tell us. It is best for you to practice twice a day for about 30 minutes each time. Now do it after me.

护士: 曾先生,不用担心。您练习的过程中我们将会对您(的情况)进行监护着。如果您有什么不适,您可以停下来并告诉我们。这个康复训练每天做两次,每次 30 分钟,您现在跟我做一遍。

Mr. Zeng: Sure, thank you.

曾先生: 好的,谢谢。

Nurse: How do you feel after practicing?

护士: 做了感觉怎样?

Mr. Zeng: It's mild, but I'm sweating a little bit.

曾先生: 动作还算柔和,但练习一遍后会微微出汗。

Nurse: You're right. The sitting version of Baduanjin is feasible for patients to practice because it contributes to circulation and organ repair. It is because the Baduanjin is a low-intensity method that the risk of **congestive heart failure** and **myocardial ischemia** would be minimized.

护士: 是的,坐式其动作简单易行,能够改善气血运行,调整脏腑功能效果显著;对体力要求较低,避免了心肌梗死后患者因剧烈运动诱发心衰、心肌缺血等不良反应。

Mr. Zeng: OK, I will do it twice a day.

曾先生: 好,那我每天坚持做两次。

(*Three days later, the patient is allowed to get out of bed.*)

(过了 3 天,患者可以下床。)

Nurse: Mr. Zeng, after practicing the sitting version of Baduanjin, you are ready to move forward to learn the standing version of it.

护士: 曾先生,这几天练习坐式八段锦,现在您可以下床,我们来练习立式八段锦。

Mr. Zeng: OK, I will give it a try.

曾先生: 好的,我来试试。

Nurse: Twice a day for 30 minutes each time. Now do it after me please.

护士: 立式您也是每天打两次,每次 30 分钟。您现在跟我一起做。

Mr. Zeng: Thanks, I can do that.

曾先生: 好,我会坚持的。

(*Two days later, Mr. Zeng is discharged.*)

（2 天后，患者可以出院）

Nurse: Mr. Zeng, how do you feel after doing Baduanjin?

护士：曾先生，进行八段锦训练后，您感觉怎样？

Mr. Zeng: I feel really comfortable and refreshed.

曾先生：一套动作下来浑身舒爽，气息顺畅。

Nurse: Wonderful! It's best for you to carry on doing the cardiac rehabilitation and we will keep following you by making a phone call once a week. Also you can call us if you have any discomfort.

护士：太好了，您回家后坚持每天这样进行心脏康复训练，我们每周会给您电话，您如果有不适可以随时给我们电话。

Mr. Zeng: Thank you very much.

曾先生：好的，谢谢您。

(*Three months later, Mr. Zeng attends the clinic.*)

（3 个月后，患者回院复诊。）

Nurse: Mr. Zeng, you look well.

护士：叔叔，精神看上去不错。

Mr. Zeng: These months, I have been practicing Baduanjin and I am making great progress. I have found that my upper body strength is increasing and it's great satisfaction for me to find that I am actually recovering, step by step.

曾先生：这几个月坚持练习八段锦，病情有很大好转，上半身力量增加了。我发现我正在逐渐康复，我也很满足现在的状态。

Nurse: According to your latest **echocardiography** report, your cardiac function also is recovering.

护士：看了您这次的心脏彩超，心功能也有很好的改善。

Mr. Zeng: Yes, I can feel it myself.

曾先生：是的，我自己也感觉到了。

Nurse: Due to its mild and progressive movements, Baduanjin is suitable for all people regardless of age and gender. It is considered as a way to strengthen your body and prevent diseases.

护士：八段锦适合男女老少平日进行锻炼，动作柔和，是递进式的动作练习，可增强体质，预防疾病。

Mr. Zeng: That's the reason why I recommend it to all my friends and my colleagues.

曾先生：是啊，我把八段锦推荐给自己的同事和亲朋好友了。

Nurse: Thank you, I am so grateful.

护士：好的，谢谢您。

Part Three　Words and Phrases

第三部分　单词和短语

circulation [ˌsɜːrkjəˈleɪʃn] *n.* 血液循环；流通，传播；发行量

【例句】Massage is used to relax muscles, relieve stress and improve the circulation. 按摩可以使肌肉放松，缓解压力和促进血液循环。

low-intensity [loʊɪntˈensɪtɪ] 低强度

【例句】Low-intensity noise can be resolved. 低强度的噪音是可以避免的。

aerobic [eˈroʊbɪk] *adj.* 需氧的，有氧的；有氧健身的，增氧健身法

【例句】Aerobic exercise gets the heart pumping and helps you to burn fat. 有氧运动加速心脏跳动，有助于消耗更多脂肪。

congestive heart failure [kənˈdʒestɪv] [haːrt] [ˈfeɪljər] 充血性心力衰竭

myocardial ischemia [ˌmaɪəˈkaːdɪrl] [ɪsˈkiːmɪr] 心肌缺血

【例句】Risk of congestive heart failure and myocardial ischemia would be minimized. 充血性心力衰竭以及心肌缺血的风险可降到最低。

echocardiography [ekoʊkaːdɪˈɒgrəfɪ] *n.* 心脏彩超

【例句】Echocardiography has been widely applied. 心脏彩超已被广泛应用。

（张晓璇）

Appendix Glossary

附 录

词汇表

A

a wide spectrum of contexts　广泛的背景

abdomen *n.* 腹部;下腹;腹腔

abdominal *adj.* 腹部的

abdominal distension　腹胀

abdominal reflex　腹壁反射

abdominal walls　腹壁

accompanied with　伴有,兼有

accumulate *vi.* 积聚;堆积

aching *adj.* 疼痛的

activating qi and collateral　益气通络

acupoint *n.* 穴道,[中医]穴位

acute *adj.* 严重的,[医]急性的;敏锐的;激烈的;
尖声的

acute myocardial infarction (AMI)　急性心肌梗死

aerobic *adj.* 需氧的,有氧的;有氧健身的,增氧健
身法

aggravate *v.* 加重

alleviate *v.* 减轻

anaphylactic *adj.* 过敏的;[医]过敏性的;导致过
敏的

angiography *n.* [特医]血管造影术;血管照相术;
血管学;[特医]血管造影法

anomalous *adj.* 异常的;不规则的

antetheca *n.* 前壁

antibiotic ointment *n.* 抗生素软膏

antibiotics *n.* [药]抗生素;抗生学

appendicitis *n.* [医]阑尾炎;盲肠炎

approximately *adv.* 大约

are separated from　与……分离

armpit *n.* 腋窝

arrange for　安排

artery *n.* 动脉;干道;主流

as follows　如下

aspiration *n.* 渴望;抱负;送气;吸气;吸引术

attempts to control bleeding　试图控制出血

auscultate *vi.* 听诊

auscultation *n.* 听诊

auxiliary *adj.* 辅助的;附加的

B

base on　基于,以……为根据

be based on ...　根据;以……为基础

be conducted by　由……指挥

be disheveled　蓬乱,凌乱

be equipped with　装用…装置;装备有

be regarded as　被认为是

be used to　习惯于;被用来做

bilateral *adj.* 双边的

bite-block *n.* 牙垫

blood sugar/ blood glucose　血糖值

blood gas analysis (ABG)　血气分析

blunt *adj.* 钝的;生硬的

blunt head trauma　头钝器伤

body parts　身体部位

bowel sound　肠鸣音

break into　突然开始

bronchitis *n.* [内科]支气管炎

bronchofibroscope *n.* 纤维支纤镜

C

cabinet *n.* 内阁;橱柜;展览艺术品的小陈列室 *adj.* 内
阁的;私下的,秘密的

cannulation *n.* 管子中空,套管插入式

cardiac *adj.* 心脏的

cardiac dullness border　心脏浊音界

cardio-cerebro-vascular　心脑血管病

catheter *n.* [医]导管;导尿管;尿液管

cefazolin sodium　头孢唑林钠

cellulose *n.* 纤维素;(植物的)细胞膜质

central *adj.* 中心的;主要的;中枢的 *n.* 电话总机

central venous catheterization *n.* 中央静脉导管置
管术

cerebral *adj.* 大脑的

cerebrovascular *adj.* 脑血管的

certified *adj.* 被证明的;有保证的;具有证明文件的

chest *n.* 胸,胸部;衣柜;箱子;金库

cholangitis *n.* 胆道炎,[内科]胆管炎

cholesterol *n.* 胆固醇

chronic obstructive pulmonary disease (COPD)
慢性阻塞性肺部疾病

circulation *n.* 血液循环;流通,传播;发行量

clench *vt.* 紧握;确定;把……敲弯 *vi.* 握紧;钉牢 *n.*
紧抓;敲环脚 *n.* (Clench)人名;(英)克伦奇

clinostatism *n.* 卧位

colic *n.* 绞痛

colonography *n.* 结肠成像术

complain of　主诉,抱怨

component *adj.* 组成的,构成的 *n.* 成分;组件;元件

computerized tomography *n.* 电脑断层摄影术

concussion *n.* 脑震荡

congestive heart failure 充血性心力衰竭

consciousness *n.* 意识

container *n.* 集装箱;容器

context *n.* 环境;上下文;来龙去脉

Continuous Positive Airway Pressure 无创呼吸机(又称持续气道正压通气)

contusion *n.* 挫伤

convention *n.* 大会;[法]惯例;约定;协定;习俗

coronary *adj.* 冠的;冠状的;花冠的;冠状动脉或静脉的

cotton swab 棉棒

CPR *abbr.* 心肺复苏术(cardiopulmonary resuscitation)

CPR certified 持有心肺复苏证明

crackle *n.* 裂纹;龟裂;爆裂声 *vt.* 使发爆裂声;使产生碎裂花纹 *vi.* 发劈啪声,发出细碎的爆裂声

cranial *adj.* 颅骨的

cranioplasty *n.* 颅骨成形术

CT scan 计算机横断面扫描(computerized tomography)

curl up 蜷起

cut down 削减;减少

cyanosis *n.* 发绀,青紫

D

deal with 处理;解决

deep vein thrombosis (DVT) 深静脉血栓形成

depressed *adj.* 沮丧的;萧条的;抑郁的

depression *n.* 沮丧;抑郁症

dextrose *n.* 葡萄糖

diagnose *vt.* 诊断;断定 *vi.* 诊断;判断

diagnosed *v.* 诊断;被诊断为(diagnose 的过去分词)

dialogue *n.* 对话;意见交换 *vi.* 对话 *vt.* 用对话表达

dialysate *n.* 透析液;渗析液

different kinds of 不同种类的,各种各样的

diffuse *adj.* 弥漫的;散开的 *vt.* 扩散;传播;漫射 *vi.* 传播;四散

disposal *n.* 处理

dizziness *n.* 头晕;头昏眼花

drainage *n.* 排水;排水系统;污水;排水面积

E

ECG *abbr.* 心电图(Electrocardiograph)

echocardiography *n.* 心脏彩超

elbow *n.* 肘部;弯头;扶手 *vt.* 推挤;用手肘推开

electrocardiograph (ECG) *n.* 心电图

electrode *n.* 电极

electrolyte disturbances 电解质紊乱

elevation *n.* 提高

emergency *n.* 紧急情况;突发事件

emesis *n.* [临床]呕吐

encephalopathy *n.* 脑病

endotracheal intubation 气管内插管

enormous *adj.* 庞大的,巨大的;凶暴的,极恶的

ethyl alcohol 酒精

exacerbation *n.* 恶化

exertion *n.* 发挥;努力;劳累

expectorate *vt.* 咳出痰;吐唾液;咯血 *vi.* 咳出痰等;吐唾液;咯血

extensive *adj.* 广泛的;大量的;广阔的

externalia *n.* 外生殖器

extubation *n.* 拔管

F

failure *n.* 失败;故障;失败者;破产

fasting *n.* 禁食

feel distended in the abdomen 腹胀

fibula *n.* 腓骨

first aid 急救、急救护理

fix one's gaze on 注视

fluid *adj.* 流动的;流畅的;不固定的 *n.* 流体;液体

fold ... around fingers 把……缠绕在手上

follow one's instruction 按照……的要求做

four diagnostic methods (inspection, auscultation and olfaction, inquiry, pulse-taking and palpation) 望闻问切

frequency of ……频率

functional condition 功能状态

formula *n.* [数]公式,准则;配方;婴儿食品

G

gastrointestinal *adj.* 胃肠的

gastrointestinal decompression 胃肠减压

gastrointestinal type 胃肠型

get dressed 穿好衣服

get up to 赶上,追上;达到

glomerulus *n.* [组织]肾小球

glucose meter 血糖仪

graphical *adj.* 图解的;绘画的

H

have a CT test CT 检查

have a huge impact on 对……有巨大影响

heart murmur 心脏杂音

hemiplegia *n.* [内科]偏瘫,半身麻痹[中医]半身不遂

hemodialysis *n.* [临床]血液透析;血液渗析

hemorrhage *n.* [病理]出血(等于 haemorrhage);番茄汁 *vt.* [病理]出血 *vi.* [病理]出血

hemorrhagic *adj.* 出血的

hospitalization *n.* 住院治疗;医院收容;住院保险(等于 hospitalization insurance)

hydrocephalus *n.* 脑积水

hydrochloride *n.* 盐酸盐;盐酸化物;氢氯化物

hygiene *n.* 卫生;卫生学;保健法

hyperglycemia *n.* 高血糖

hypoglycemia *n.* 低血糖

I

ICU　重症监护室（intensive care unit）

immerse ... in water　把……浸到水里

in accordance with　依照；与……一致

in addition to　除……之外

in charge of　负责；主管

in order to ...　为了……

indicate *vt.* 表明；指出；预示；象征

infarction *n.* 梗塞；［病理］梗塞形成，梗死形成

infusion *n.* 输液；输注；灌输；浸泡

inhalation *n.* 吸入；吸入药剂

insert *vt.* 插入；刺入；进针

inserted *adj.* 插入的；［生物］嵌入的；著生的；附着的

insertion *n.* 插入；嵌入；插入物

inspection *n.* ［中医］望诊

institution *n.* 制度；建立；公共机构；习俗

insufficiency *n.* 不足，不充分；功能不全；不适当

insulin *n.* 胰岛素

Intensive Care Unit (ICU)　重症监护室

intercostal *adj.* 肋间的

interference *n.* 干扰，冲突

intracerebral *adj.* 大脑内的

intracutaneous *adj.* 皮内的

intracutaneous injection　皮内注射

intravenous *adj.* 静脉内的

intravenous infusion　静脉输液

intubation *n.* ［临床］插管

inversion *n.* 倒置；反向

ipsilateral *adj.* 身体的同侧的

K

keep ... from　免于……，避免……

L

LDL=low density lipoprotein *n.* 低密度脂蛋白

lead　导联

lie on your side　翻身

lipitor *n.* 立普妥（药品名，降血脂药）

listless *adj.* 倦怠的；无精打采的

low-intensity　低强度

lymph *n.* 淋巴

M

made up of　由……组成；由……构成

medication *n.* 药物；药物治疗

monitor *v.* 监控；监听；监测 *n.* 监控器

monitoring *n.* 监视，［自］监控；检验，检查 *v.* 监视，［通信］［军］监听，监督（monitor 的 ing 形式）

motor function　运动功能

MRI　核磁共振（magnetic resonance imaging）

murmur *n.* 低语；低语声

muscle strength　肌力

myocardial *adj.* 心肌的

myocardial ischemia　心肌缺血

N

nausea *n.* 恶心

nauseate *vi.* 作呕；厌恶；产生恶感 *vt.* 使厌恶；使恶心；使作呕

necrosis *n.* 坏死；坏疽；骨疽

NG tube = nasal gastric tube　鼻胃管

nitroglycerin *n.* 硝酸甘油；硝化甘油

no matter what　无论怎么

noninvasive *adj.* 非侵袭的；非侵害的

NPO［拉丁语］（=nothing by mouth）　禁饮食

O

observation *n.* 观察

olive *n.* 橄榄，橄榄树

oral *adj.* 口头的，口述的 *n.* 口试；(Oral) 人名；（土）奥拉尔

osteogenesisimperfectan *n.* 成骨不全症

oxygen *n.* 氧气

P

painkiller *n.* 止痛药

palpation *n.* 触诊

palpitation *n.* 心悸

pancreases *n.* 胰腺

pancreatic juice *n.* 胰液

pancreatitis *n.* ［内科］胰腺炎

pelvic *adj.* 骨盆的

penicillin *n.* 青霉素

per *prep.* 每；经；按照；每一 *n.* (Per) 人名；（德、挪、丹、瑞典）佩尔

percussion *n.* 叩诊

percutaneons *adj.* 经皮的；经由皮肤的

perforation *n.* 穿孔；贯穿

peristaltic wave　蠕动波

peritonitis *n.* ［内科］腹膜炎

pin care *n.* 钢针（牵引用）护理

plaque *n.* 斑块

plavix *n.* 氯吡格雷（波立维）

play an integral role　扮演着不可或缺的角色

pneumothorax *n.* 气胸

post-op *adj.* ［口语］=postoperative　手术后

precordium *n.* 心前区，心窝

progressive *adj.* 进步的；先进的 *n.* 改革论者；进步分子

promoting circulation and removing stasis　活血化瘀

proximal *adj.* 最接近的，邻近的；近身体中央的

pulmonary *adj.* 肺的；有肺的；肺状的

pulse-taking *n.* ［中医］脉诊

pump *v.* 泵入

put aside　把……放在一边

put on　戴上

R

radiating *adj.* 发射出（光、热等）（radiate 的现在分词）*v.*（使品质或情感）显出，流露；射出，向四周伸出；散热

radiographic *adj.* 射线照相术的

reference *n.* 参考,参照;涉及,参考书目;介绍信;证明书

rehabilitation *n.* 康复,复原

renal *adj.* [解剖]肾脏的,[解剖]肾的 *n.* (Renal)人名;(法)勒纳尔

respiratory *adj.* 呼吸的

retrosternal *adj.* 胸骨后的

right heart failure 右心衰竭

S

sacrum *n.* [解剖]骶骨;[解剖]荐骨

sample *vt.* 取样;尝试;抽样检查 *n.* 样品;样本;例子;(Sample)人名;(英)桑普尔 *adj.* 试样的,样品的;作为例子的

saturated with ... 浸透……

saturation *n.* 饱和;色饱和度;浸透;磁化饱和

semi-permeable *adj.* 半渗透的

sensation *n.* 感觉

septic *adj.* 败血症的;[医]脓毒性的;腐败的 *n.* 腐烂物

severe pancreatitis 重症胰腺炎

shifting dullness 移动性浊音

short of breath 呼吸短促

shortness of breath 气促;呼吸浅短

skeletal *adj.* 骨骼的,像骨骼的;骸骨的;骨瘦如柴的

sleeve *n.* [机]套筒,套管;袖子,[服装]袖套 *vt.* 给……装袖子;给……装套筒

smear *v.* 涂抹

soak *vt.* 吸收,吸入;沉浸在(工作或学习中);使……上下湿透 *vi.* 浸泡;渗透 *n.* 浸;湿透;大雨

spectrum *n.* 光谱;频谱;范围;余象

spit into ... 吐出到……

sputum *n.* [生理]痰;唾液

squeezing *adj.* 挤压的;压榨的

stable *adj.* 稳定的

stent *n.* [医]斯滕特氏印模膏;支架;展伸;(Stent)人名;(英)斯滕特 *adj.* 扩张的

sterilize *vt.* 消毒,杀菌;使成不毛;使绝育;使不起作用

stethoscope *n.* 听诊器

stomach *n.* 胃;腹部;胃口

stomachache *n.* 腹痛

stuffy *adj.* 闷热的;古板的;不通气的

subclavian vein *n.* 锁骨下静脉

subcutaneous varicose vein 静脉曲张

sublingual *adj.* 舌下的;舌下腺的

sublingually *adj.* 舌下的;舌下腺的

suction *n.* 吸;吸力;抽吸

suffer from 忍受;遭受;患……病;受……苦

suppurative *adj.* 化脓的;化脓性的;使化脓的 *n.* 吸脓药;化脓促进剂

surgical *adj.* 外科的;手术上的 *n.* 外科手术;外科病房

swallow *vi.* 吞下;咽下

sweating *v.* 出汗(sweat 的 ing 形式)*n.* 发汗(等于 exudation)

swelling *n.* 肿胀;膨胀;增大;涨水 *adj.* 膨胀的;肿大的;突起的 *v.* 肿胀;膨胀;增多;趾高气扬(swell 的 ing 形式)

symmetric *adj.* 对称的;匀称的

syringe *n.* 注射器;洗涤器

syrup *n.* 含药糖浆,果汁

T

tablet *n.* 药片,小片

take off 脱掉

teaspoonful *n.* 一茶匙的量

the former 前者

the majority of ……的大多数(反义词 minority)

therapeutic *adj.* 治疗的;治疗学的;有益于健康的;*n.* 治疗剂;治疗学家

therapist *n.* 临床医学家;治疗学家

therapy *n.* 治疗,疗法

thermometer *n.* 温度计;体温计

thorax *n.* 胸;胸腔

thrombosis *n.* [病理]血栓形成;血栓症

thyroid *n.* 甲状腺

tibia *n.* 胫骨

tidal volumn *n.* 潮气肺容物

trachea *n.* 气管

trauma *n.* [外科]创伤

treatment *n.* 治疗

troubleshooting *n.* 解决纷争;发现并修理故障 *v.* 检修(troubleshoot 的 ing 形式);当调解人

tube *n.* 管;电子管;隧道;电视机 *vt.* 使成管状;把…装管;用管输送 *vi.* 乘地铁;不及格

turn blue 发青紫

tympanitic note 鼓音

U

ultrafiltration *n.* [化学]超滤,[环境]超滤作用

umbilicus *n.* 脐,种脐;中心

upheaval *n.* 隆起

urine *n.* 尿

V

vascular *adj.* 血管的

venous *adj.* 静脉的;有脉纹的

ventilation *n.* 通风设备;空气流通

ventilator *n.* 通风设备;换气扇;【医】呼吸机

verification *n.* 确认,查证;核实

vital *adj.* 至关重要的;生死攸关的;有活力的

vital sign 生命体征

vomit *n. v.* 呕吐

vomiting *v.* 呕吐(vomit 的 ing 形式)

W

waveform *n.* [物][电子]波形

wring thoroughly 彻底绞干

参考文献

［1］高燕. 护理专业英语. 北京：人民卫生出版社，2015.

［2］刘红霞. 护理专业英语. 北京：中国中医药出版社，2013.

［3］谷岩梅. 护理专业英语. 北京：人民卫生出版社，2009.

［4］Craig Louey. 西方临床护理英语全攻略. 北京：北京大学医学出版社，2007.

［5］余雪. 护理专业英语. 北京：化学工业出版社，2015.

［6］徐淑秀，李建群. 实用护理英语. 北京：人民军医出版社，2009.

［7］Perry J，蔡碧华. 护理美语. 北京：科学出版社，2006.

［8］强力宁，杨潇潇. 护理英语. 北京：人民军医出版社，2014.

［9］侯惠如. 护理病例荟萃. 北京：人民军医出版社，2011.

［10］朗文当代高级英语词典. 北京：商务印书馆，1998.

［11］才秀颖. 涉外医疗及护理英语. 北京：军事医学科学出版社，2009.

［12］李红，林惠珠. 重症医学专科护士实践手册. 北京：化学工业出版社，2013.

［13］张伟英. 实用重症医学监护护理. 上海：上海科学技术出版社，2005.

［14］张洪君. 当代临床专科护理操作手册. 北京：人民军医出版社，2006.

［15］王文秀，王颖. 英汉对照护理英语会话. 北京：人民卫生出版社，2011.

［16］亚当. 实用医学英语会话. 北京：中国水利水电出版社，2007.

［17］张玲芝. 实用护理英语. 杭州：浙江大学出版社，2010.

［18］Di S E, Tartaglini D, Fiorini S, et al. Medication errors in intensive care units: nurses' training needs. Emergency Nurse the Journal of the Rcn Accident & Emergency Nursing Association, 2016, 24(4): 24–29.

［19］H Minami. Implementation of a multicomponent process to obtain informed consent in the Diabetes Control and Complications Trial. The DCCT Research Group. Controlled Clinical Trials,1989, 10 (1) : 83–96.

［20］TD Group. Intensive diabetes therapy and glomerular filtration rate in type 1 diabetes. New England Journal of Medicine, 2011, 365 (25): 2366.

［21］LS Perrin. Preventing complications of central venous catheterization. New England Journal of Medicine, 2003, 348 (26): 2684.

［22］Cruzeiro, PAM Camargos, ME Miranda. Central venous catheter placement in children:

a prospective study of complications in a Brazilian public hospital. Pediatric Surgery International, 2006, 22 (6): 536–540.

［23］RRTS Investigators, R Bellomo, A Cass, et al. Intensity of continuous renal-replacement therapy in critically ill patients. New England Journal of Medicine, 2009, 361 (17): 1627.

［24］H Schiffl. The dark side of high-intensity renal replacement therapy of acute kidney injury in critically ill patients. International Urology and Nephrology, 2010, 42 (2) : 435–440.

［25］L Nilsson, A Johansson, S Kalman. Monitoring of respiratory rate in postoperative care using a new photoplethysmographic technique. Journal of Clinical Monitoring and Computing, 2000, 16 (4): 309–315.

［26］Nilsson L, Johansson A, Kalman S. Monitoring of respiratory rate in postoperative care using a new photoplethysmographic technique. Journal of Clinical Monitoring & Computing, 2000, 16 (4): 309–315.

［27］RM Wachter, KG Shojania, AJ Markowitz, et al. Quality grand rounds: the case for patient safety. Annals of Internal Medicine, 2006, 145 (8): 629–630.

［28］DL Elliot, DH Hickam. Attending rounds on in-patient units: differences between medical and non-medical services. Medical Education, 1993, 27 (6) : 503 – 508.

［29］AC Estes, M Asce, MF Dan, et al. Updating bridge reliability based on bridge management systems visual inspection results. Journal of Bridge Engineering, 2003, 8 (6): 374–382.

［30］Dan M. Frangopol, Min Liu. Maintenance and management of civil infrastructure based on condition, safety, optimization, and life-cycle cost. Structure & Infrastructure Engineering, 2007, 3 (1): 29–41.

［31］NIOC Health. The relation of child care to cognitive and language development. Child Development, 2000, 71 (4) : 960.